Grizzly 399

The Story of a Remarkable Bear

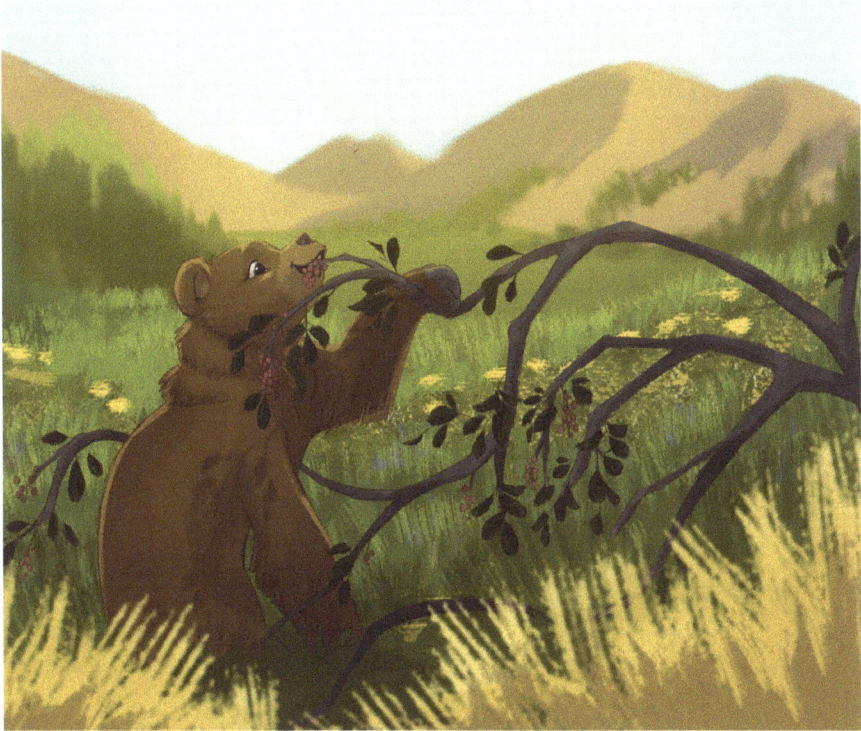

By Sylvia M. Medina

Photography by Thomas D. Mangelsen

Illustrations by Morgan Spicer

green kids club

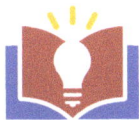

NoahText®

Noah Text®

The **Noah Text®** Chapter Books have been carefully selected and curated to meet the needs of all readers – and striving and struggling readers in particular – by providing superior text accessibility. Noah Text® books are rendered in **Noah Text®, a patented evidence-based methodology for displaying text that increases reading skill.**

Grounded in the science of reading, Noah Text® is a specialized scaffolded text that shows **syllable patterns** within words by highlighting them with bold and unbold and marking **long vowels** (vowels that "say their own names"). Here are some examples:

entertainment	⇨	**en**ter**tain**ment
beautiful	⇨	**beau**tiful
photosynthesis	⇨	**pho**to**syn**the**sis**
comprehension	⇨	**com**pre**hen**sion
ironic	⇨	i**ron**ic
lieutenant	⇨	**lieu**ten**ant**
achievement	⇨	a**chieve**ment
epitome	⇨	e**pit**ome
ideology	⇨	i**de**ol**ogy**
coordination	⇨	**co**or**di**na**tion**

By showing readers the structure of words, Noah Text® enhances reading skills, freeing up cognitive resources that readers can devote to comprehension. Noah Text® simulates simpler writing systems (e.g., Finland's) in which learning to read is easier due to visible, predictable word patterns. As a result, Noah Text® increases reading fluency, stamina, accuracy, and confidence while building skills that transfer to plain text reading.

Highly recommended by structured literacy specialists, Noah Text® is effective for developing, struggling, and dyslexic readers and for multilingual learners. Noah Text® enables resistant and struggling readers to advance their reading skills beyond basic proficiency so that they can tackle higher-level learning.

Readers find Noah Text® intuitive and easy to use, requiring little to no instruction to get started. A sound key that further explains how Noah Text® works can be found at the back of this book.

For further information on Noah Text® and its products, please visit www.noahtext.com.

Dear Parents, Educators, and Striving English-Language Readers,

As individuals develop the ability to read beyond the elementary level, their challenge is to build on a basic awareness of how patterns of letters stand for sounds and how those sounds come together to make words. Readers who learn the letter patterns in one-syllable words are poised to recognize them in longer, multisyllable words.

For struggling readers, however, long words can appear to be a sea of individual letters whose syllable sub-divisions are hard to discern. This s eries from Noah Text® highlights where syllable breaks occur, while also signaling long vowels -- those that "say their own names."   These visual cues help struggling readers decode words more easily and read more fluently and accurately.

Now, with Noah Text® Chapter Books, all individuals can learn to read with less effort, empowering them to experience enriching l iterature and enlightening informational texts.

Miriam Cherkes-Julkowski, Ph.D.
Professor, Educational Psychology (retired)
Educational Diagnostician and Consultant

About the Author - Sylvia M. Medina is the president, primary author, and creative director of the Green Kids Club. She has spent her career focused on environmental issues and helping to preserve animal welfare. She developed the Green Kids Club concept, which would help her children, as well as other children around the world, learn early positive environmental habits that they could share with others.

About the Photographer
Thomas D. Mangelsen is an American nature and wildlife photographer and conservationist. He is most famous for his photography of wildlife in the Greater Yellowstone Ecosystem. He has been active in the movement to keep the Yellowstone area grizzly bears on the Endangered Species List.

About the Illustrator – Morgan Spicer is the founder of Bark Point Studio. She lives a vegan life in NJ, with her 6 rescue dogs and husband. Morgan has illustrated over 40 books and has created thousands of custom portraits since graduating from Syracuse University in 2012.

Contributors - Louisa Willcox , Grace Peters, Shelley Mascia, Joy Eagle

green kids club
www.greenkidsclub.com

Grizzly 399

The Story of a Remarkable Bear

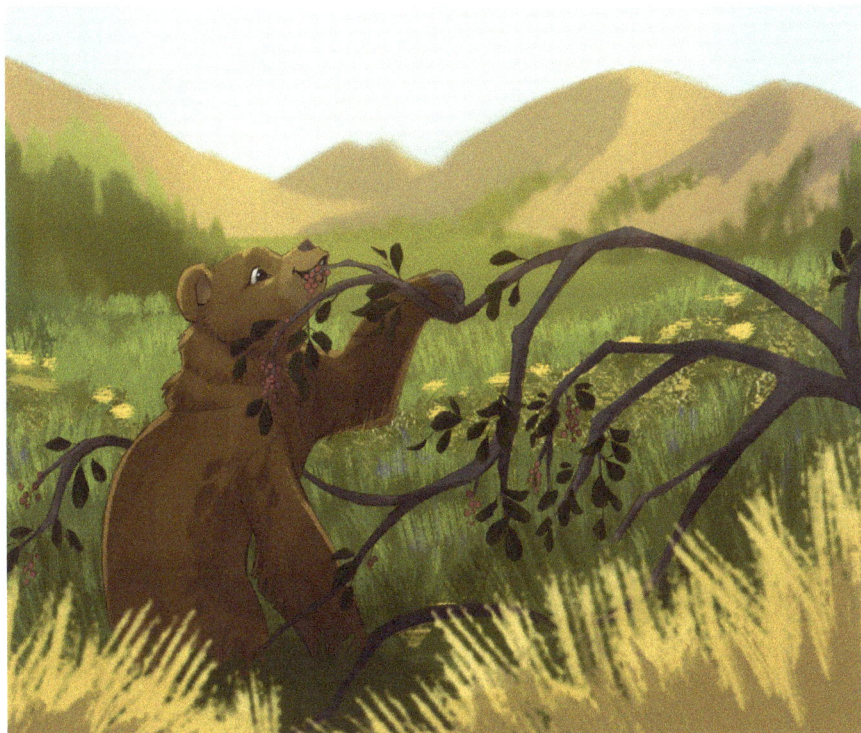

By Sylvia M. Medina

Photography by Thomas D. Mangelsen

Illustrations by Morgan Spicer

green kids club

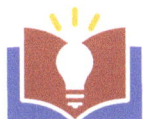

Noah Text

CONTENTS

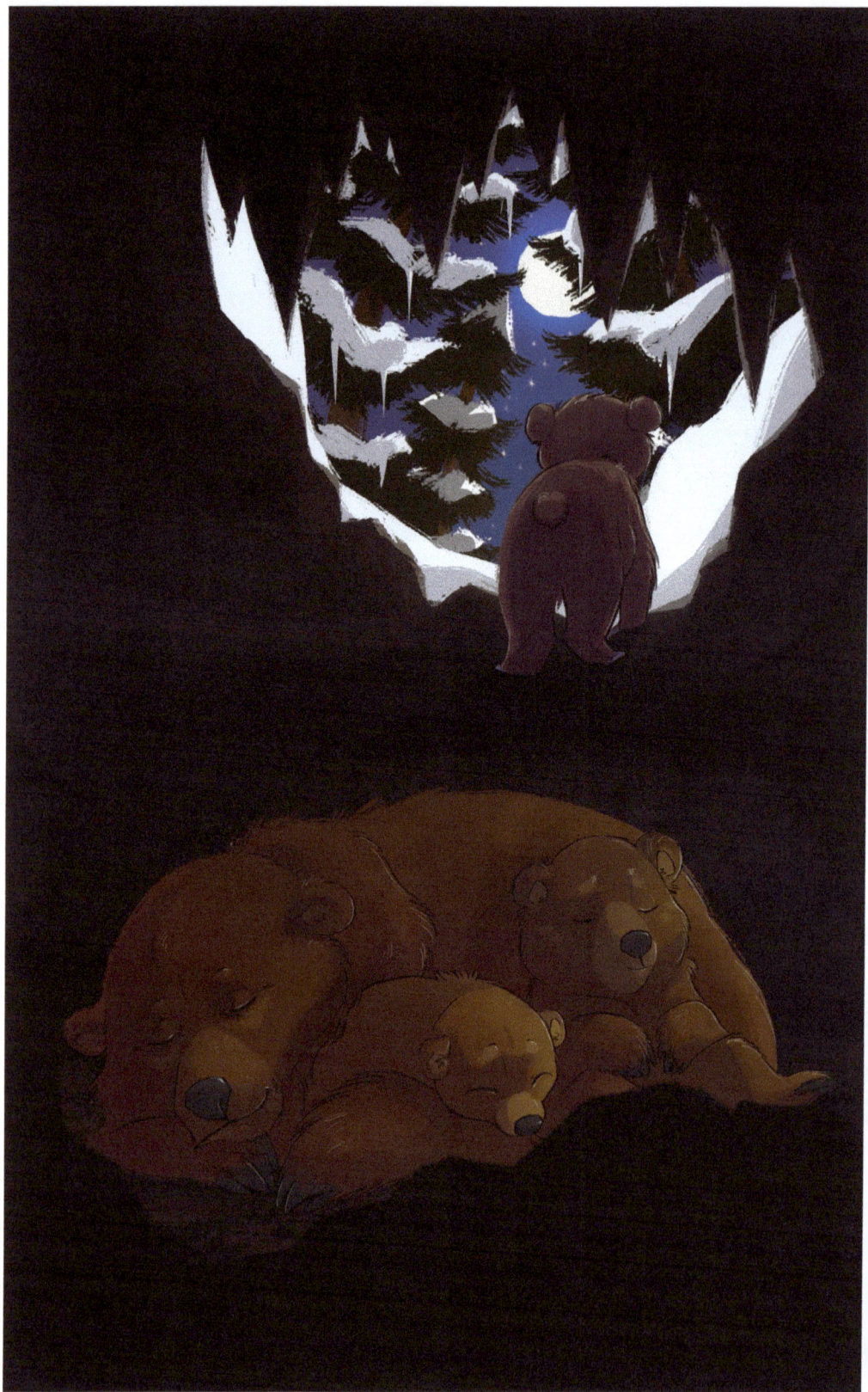

M<u>ee</u>t **Sis**ter Be<u>a</u>r

It was dark in the c<u>a</u>ve where **B<u>a</u>**by Be<u>a</u>r, or "**Sis**ter Be<u>a</u>r" as sh<u>e</u> was called, was **sleep**ing. Sh<u>e</u> was **cud**dled up **a**gainst her **moth**er and two **broth**ers, "**Lit**tle Cub" and "Big Cub," who were all **snor**ing **loud**ly. **Swish**ing sounds c<u>a</u>me from the c<u>a</u>ve's <u>o</u>pen**ing**. **Sis**ter Be<u>a</u>r was s<u>o</u> c<u>o</u>zy and warm, **snug**gled up **a**gainst her **moth**er's thick c<u>o</u>at, but **cu**ri**osity** got the best of her. Sh<u>e</u> **sl<u>o</u>w**ly got up and crept **to**ward the soft gl<u>o</u>w at the mouth of the c<u>a</u>ve.

Sister Be<u>a</u>r p<u>ee</u>ked **out**s<u>i</u>de and sniffed the c<u>o</u>ld <u>a</u>ir. **Look**ing **a**round, sh<u>e</u> saw that the world was **cov**ered in a **fluff**y, wh<u>i</u>te **blan**ket. Sh<u>e</u> took two **care**ful steps out of the c<u>a</u>ve. When her **fur**ry paws sank **in**to the sn<u>o</u>w, sh<u>e</u> jumped back. It's c<u>o</u>ld! sh<u>e</u> thought.

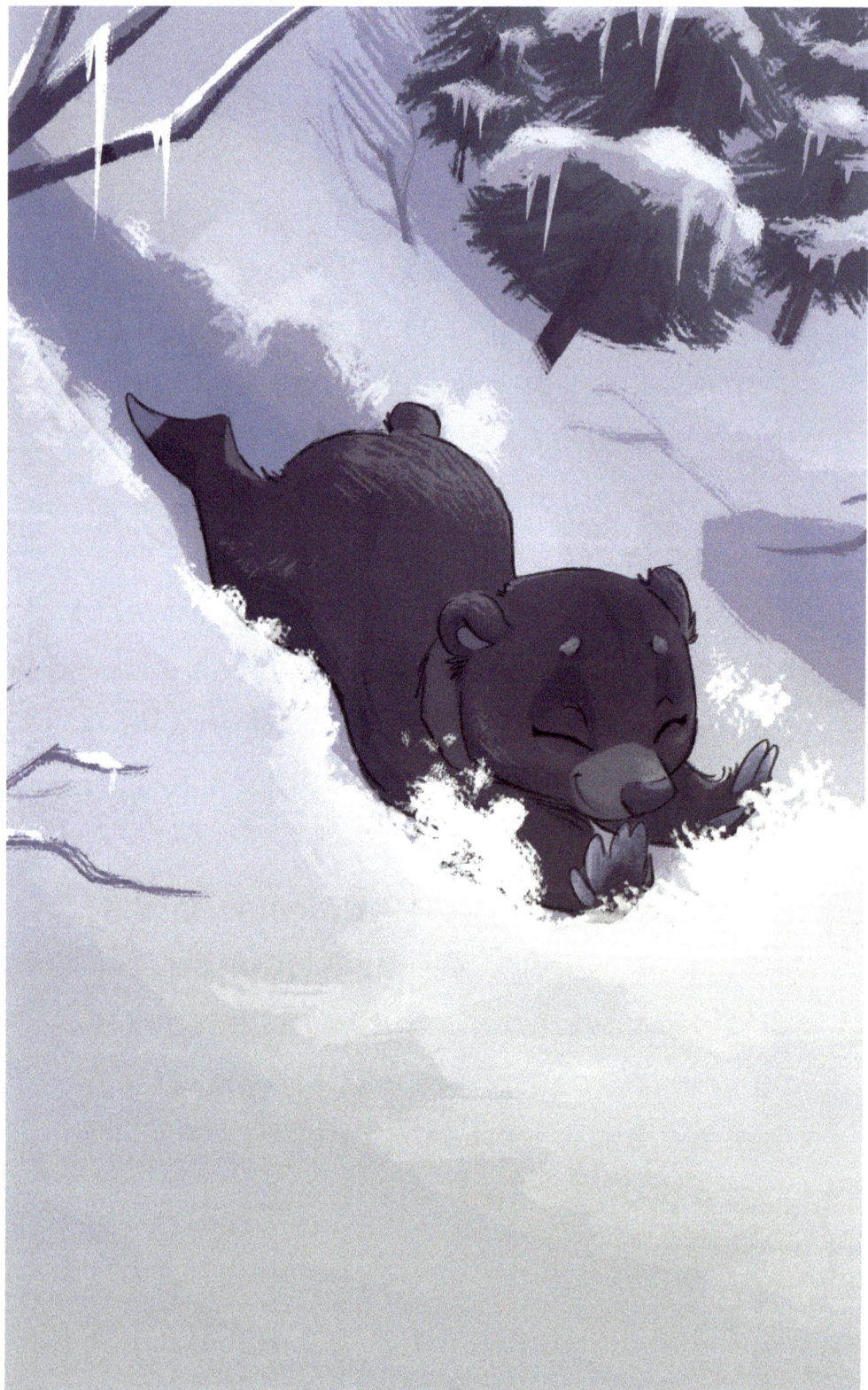

Sister Be__a__r looked down at the tr__ee__-**cov**ered sl__o__pe which **spar**kled in the **moon**light. **Sud**den**ly**, sh__e__ had an __i__d__e__**a**. **Bolt**ing from the c__a__ve, sh__e__ ran down the hill as fast as sh__e__ could, **kick**ing up a cloud of wh__i__te **pow**der as sh__e__ **bound**ed down the slope. **Half**w__a__y down, she **stum**bled __o__ver a sn__o__w-**cov**ered rock and r__o__lled the rest of the w__a__y to the **bot**tom.

Whumpf! Sh__e__ **land**ed in a d__ee__p sn__o__w drift.

Her **moth**er and **broth**ers w__o__ke up and c__a__me **run**ning down the hill **af**ter her. Her **broth**ers r__o__lled and **tum**bled **b__e__**hind her **moth**er, who was **sl__o__w**ly **l__o__p**ing **a**long down the hill with a stern look on her f__a__ce.

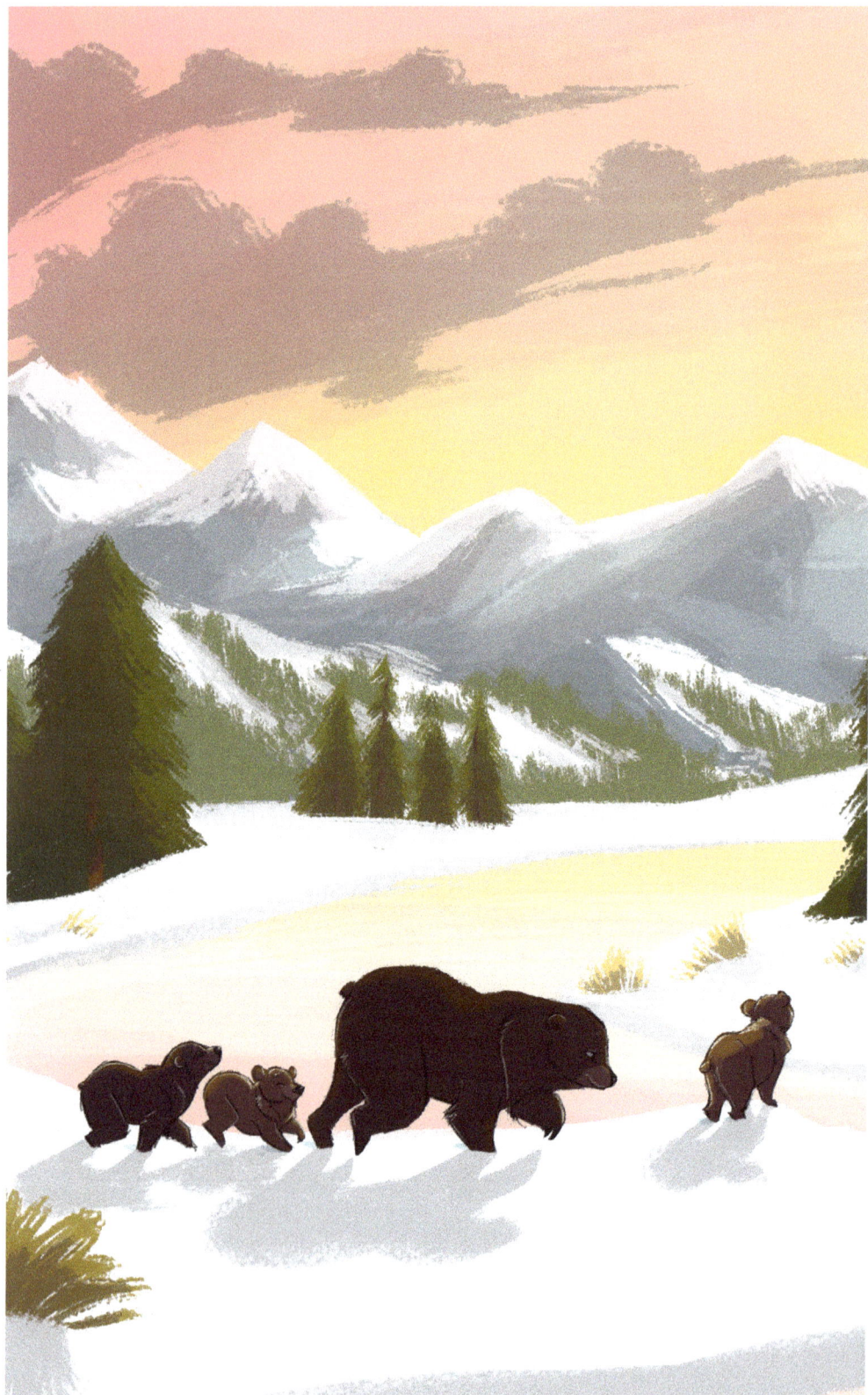

"Now you've done it!" her **moth**er said. "We have to climb all the way back up to our den!" Her **moth**er paused and looked **a**round. She sighed. "Well, we're down here—I might as well show you some of your new world!"

As the sky turned pink and gold, her **moth**er led them through the **wood**lands to a wide, **rush**ing stream. She took a drink and then **mo**tioned for them to do the same. **Some**thing caught her eye, and she pounced. From out of the stream, she pulled a large fish, a **Rain**bow Trout. It **glis**tened in the **morn**ing sun as she held it in her great, **pow**er**ful** jaws. She dropped it in front of **Sis**ter Bear and her **broth**ers.

She took a small bite and then nudged it **to**ward **Ba**by Bear. "Eat!" **Moth**er said.

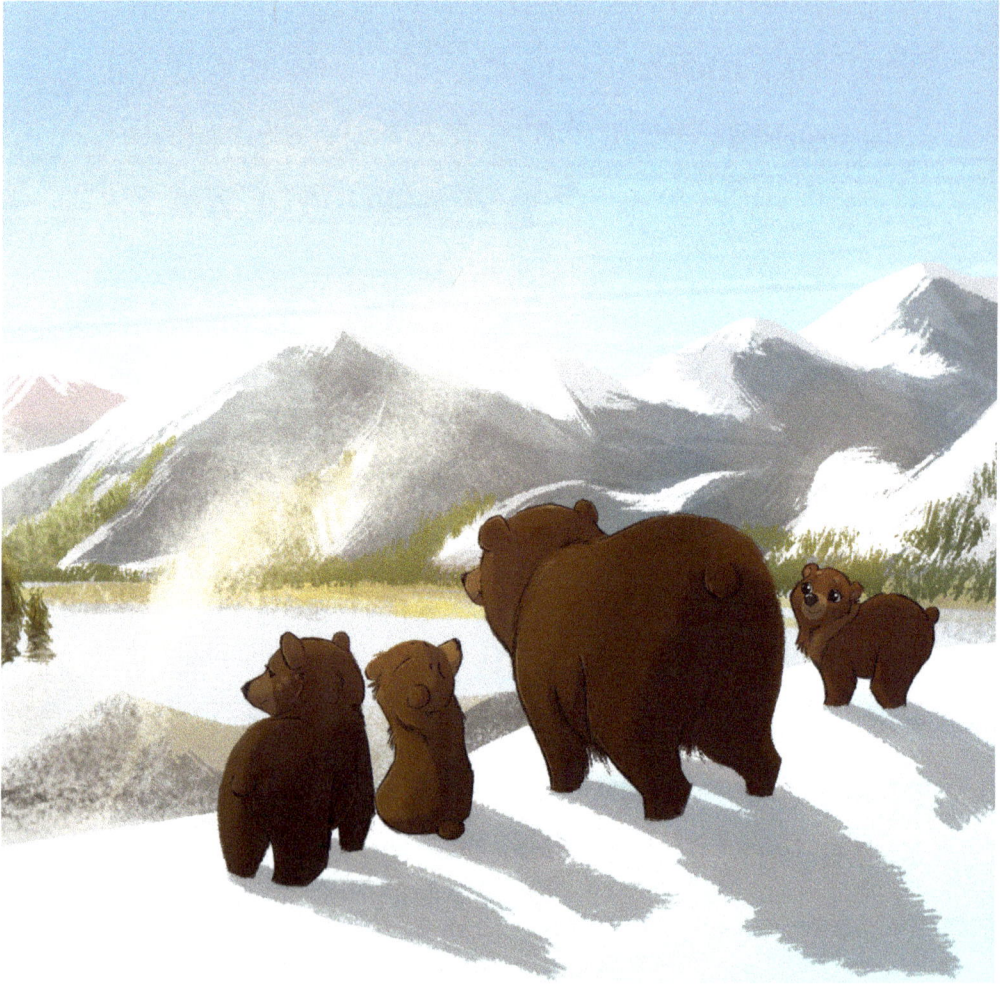

Sister Be<u>a</u>r and her **broth**ers took turns t<u>a</u>king b<u>i</u>tes of **de**licious fish.

After **break**fast, their **moth**er led them to some **gey**sers: **st<u>ea</u>m**ing pits that spr<u>a</u>yed w<u>a</u>ter from the ground. "Th<u>e</u>se are hot!" **Moth**er said. "St<u>ay</u> **a**w<u>ay</u> from th<u>e</u>se!"

They **wan**dered on and soon c<u>a</u>me to a **moun**tain. The young cubs **fol**l<u>o</u>wed their **moth**er up the st<u>ee</u>p sl<u>o</u>pe. When they got to the top, **Moth**er looked off in the **dis**tance **to**ward a gre<u>a</u>t **moun**tain r<u>a</u>nge. Th<u>o</u>se are the **tall**est things <u>I</u>'ve **ev**er s<u>ee</u>n! thought **B<u>a</u>**by Be<u>a</u>r.

"Look, **chil**dren," **Moth**er said. "**Some**d<u>ay</u>, yo<u>u</u> m<u>a</u>y want to g<u>o</u> live in th<u>o</u>se gre<u>a</u>t **moun**tains. There are str<u>ea</u>ms full of fish, yo<u>u</u> can **al**s<u>o</u> hunt elk or **for**age for sw<u>ee</u>t **ber**ri<u>e</u>s."

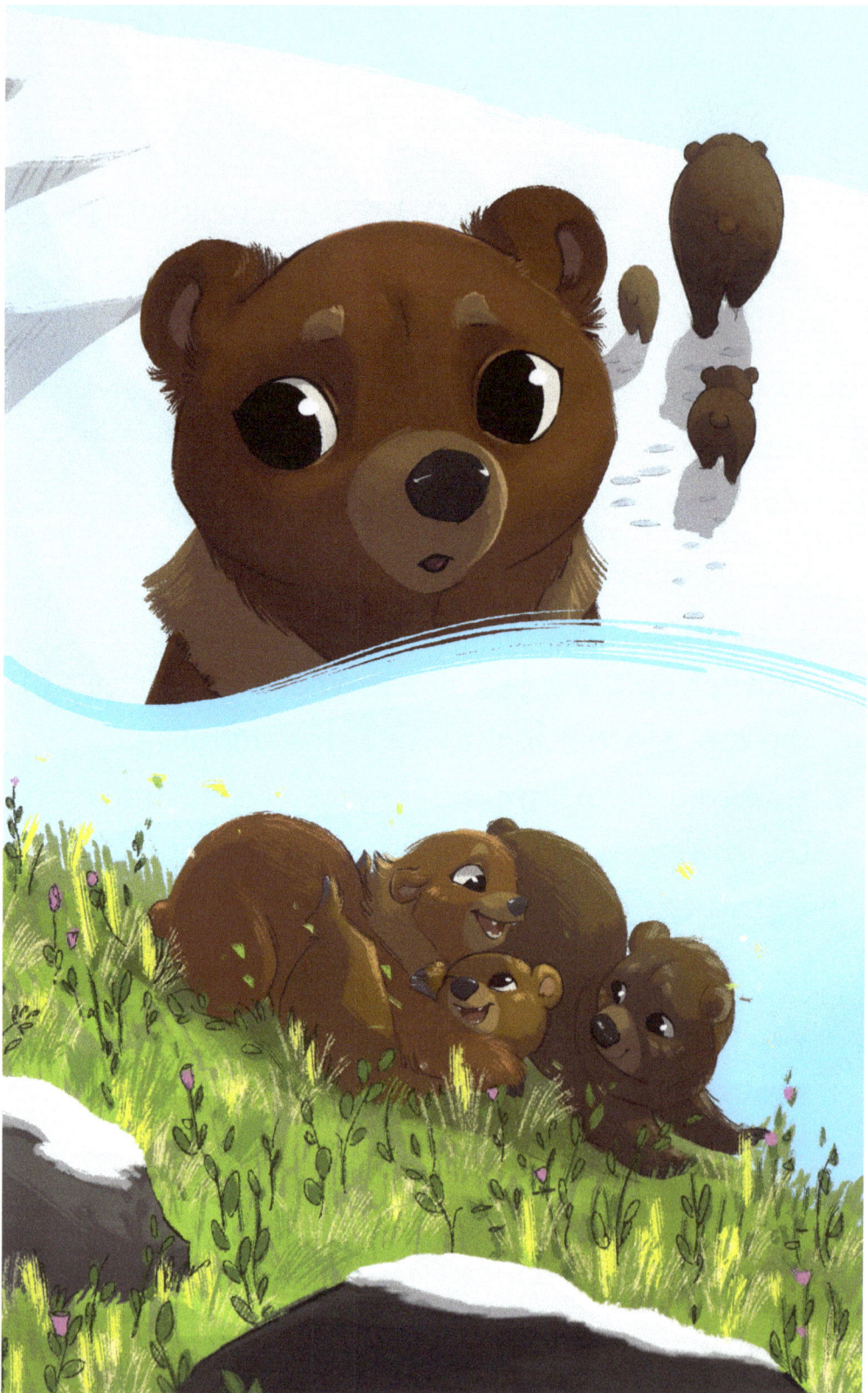

Sister Be<u>a</u>r looked at the far **a**w<u>ay</u>, sn<u>o</u>w-capped p<u>ea</u>ks.

Sh<u>e</u> **could**n't **ima**g**ine cl<u>i</u>mb**ing s<u>o</u> h<u>i</u>gh or **liv**ing s<u>o</u> far from her **fam**ily.

"Let's g<u>o</u> back to the den and get some rest," her **moth**er said. They **r<u>e</u>**turned to the c<u>a</u>ve to w<u>ai</u>t for spring.

Spring **f<u>i</u>**nal**ly** **ar**r<u>i</u>ved and the Be<u>a</u>r **fam**ily <u>e</u>merged from their den. M<u>o</u>st of the sn<u>o</u>w had **melt**ed and the world looked fresh and gr<u>ee</u>n. **Sis**ter Be<u>a</u>r, **Lit**tle Cub, and Big Cub romped thro<u>u</u>gh w<u>i</u>de **mead<u>o</u>ws, r<u>o</u>ll**ing and **pl<u>ay</u>**ing **a**mong the **bud**ding **w<u>i</u>ld**flow**ers**.

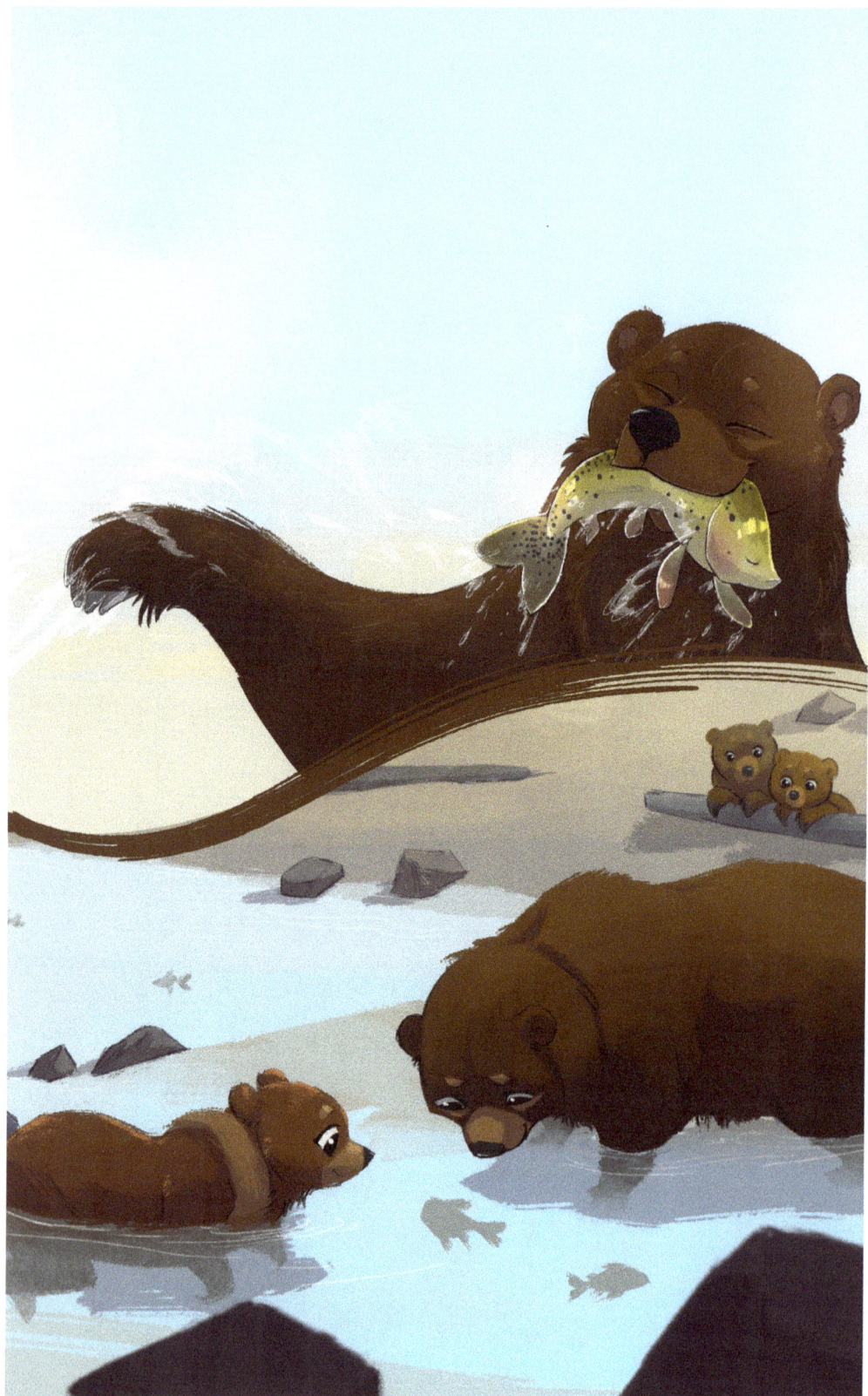

Mother led them to the str<u>ea</u>m once more and taught the cubs to fish. Sh<u>e</u> **al**s<u>o</u> taught them to hunt for elk and d<u>ee</u>r.

T<u>i</u>me passed and as spring **be**c<u>a</u>me **sum**mer, the cubs r<u>oa</u>med the **moun**tains and **for**ests with their **moth**er, **hunt**ing, **fish**ing, <u>ea</u>ting, and **pl<u>ay</u>**ing. The **lit**tle be<u>a</u>rs were **gr<u>o</u>w**ing fast!

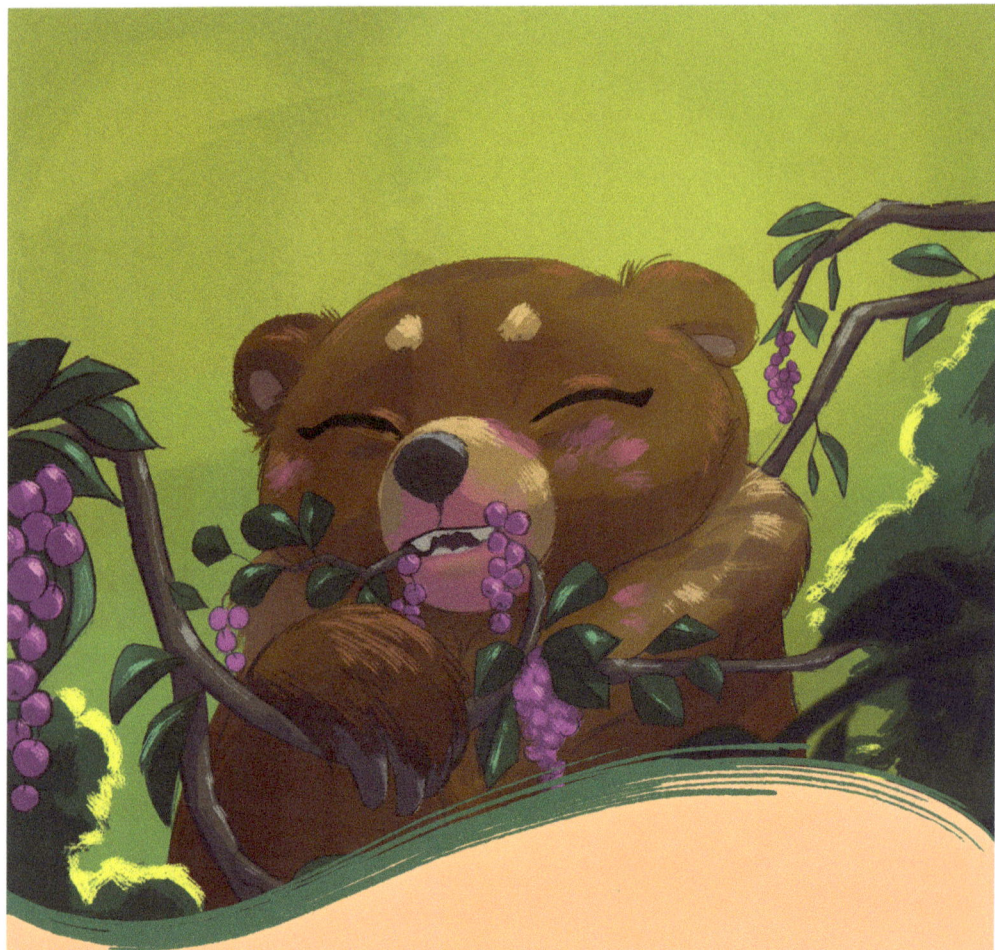

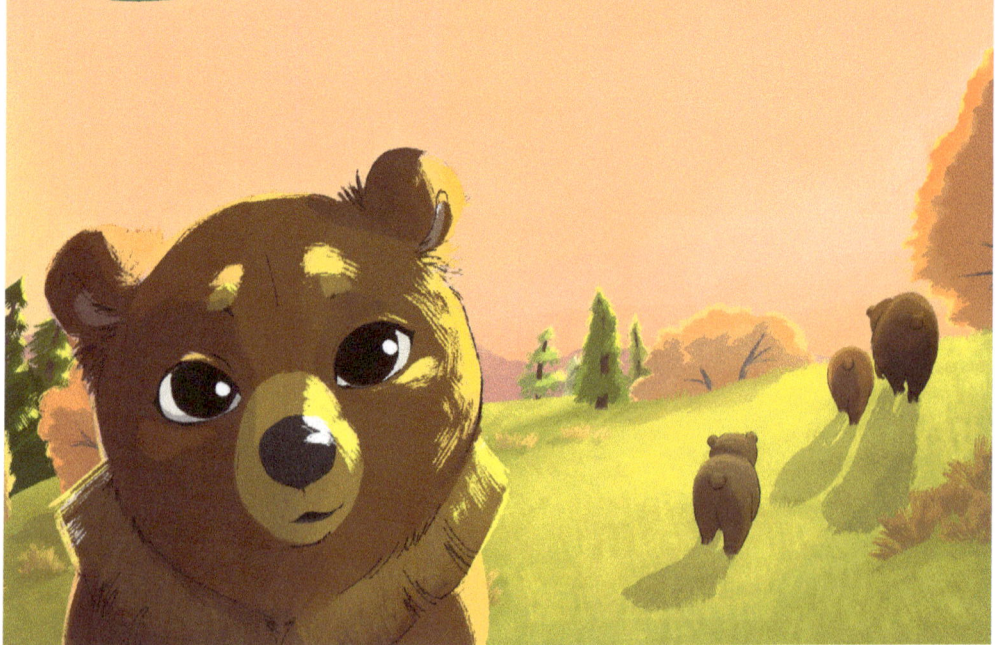

One d<u>ay</u> in the **earl**y fall, **Moth**er took them **in**to the woods and sh<u>ow</u>ed them some **bush**es full of sw<u>ee</u>t, **ju**icy **huck**leber<u>rie</u>s. As the cubs <u>a</u>te the **ber**ri<u>es</u>, their **muz**zles **turn**ing red and **pur**ple, **Moth**er said, "Fill your **tum**mi<u>es</u>, kids, for yo<u>u</u> n<u>eed</u> to <u>e</u>at a lot! **Win**ter is **com**ing soon!"

Several d<u>ay</u>s l<u>at</u>er, they **be**gan the long trek back up to their den. **Sis**ter Bear looked off at the far **aw<u>ay</u>** **moun**tain r<u>a</u>nge as they **plod**ded **a**long. Sh<u>e</u> was **c<u>u</u>rious** to s<u>ee</u> the pl<u>a</u>ce **Moth**er had **de**scr<u>i</u>bed. The be<u>a</u>rs went **in**to the c<u>a</u>ve to **h<u>i</u>**ber**n<u>a</u>te** and w<u>ai</u>t out the long, c<u>o</u>ld **win**ter.

When spring c<u>a</u>me **a**gain, **Sis**ter Bear's **moth**er led the cubs to the str<u>ea</u>m once more. Sh<u>e</u> sat down and looked at them **thought**fully.

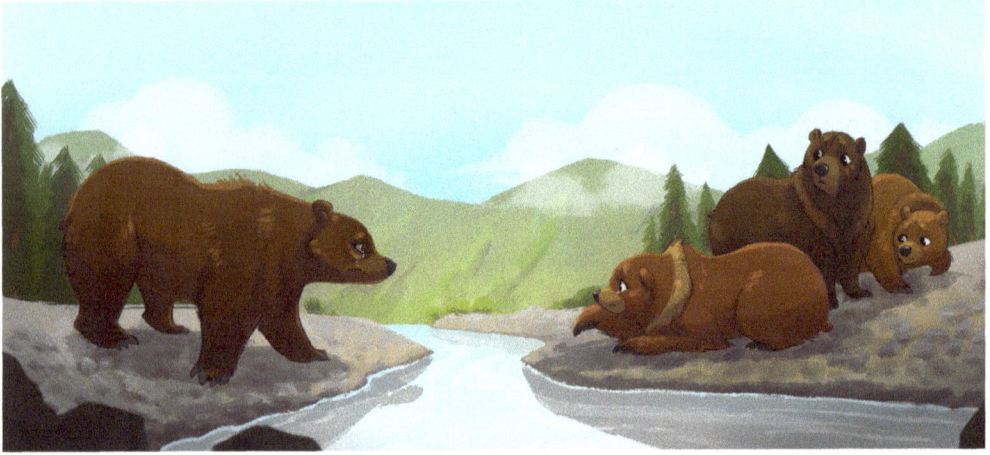

"You all have grown so much! You are **get**ting to be great, big bears! It's time for you to go out on your own, now."

But **Ma**ma!" **Sis**ter Bear cried."We're still your **ba**bies! We want to stay with you!"

Little Cub and Big Cub **be**gan to moan and whine and shake their **fur**ry heads.

"I am **go**ing now," their **moth**er growled **firm**ly. "You **can**not **fol**low me. You must make your own way in the world now."

Sister Bear and her **broth**ers sat by the stream and watched their **moth**er walk **a**way. Tears rolled down her snout as she watched her **moth**er **dis**ap**pear in**to the trees.

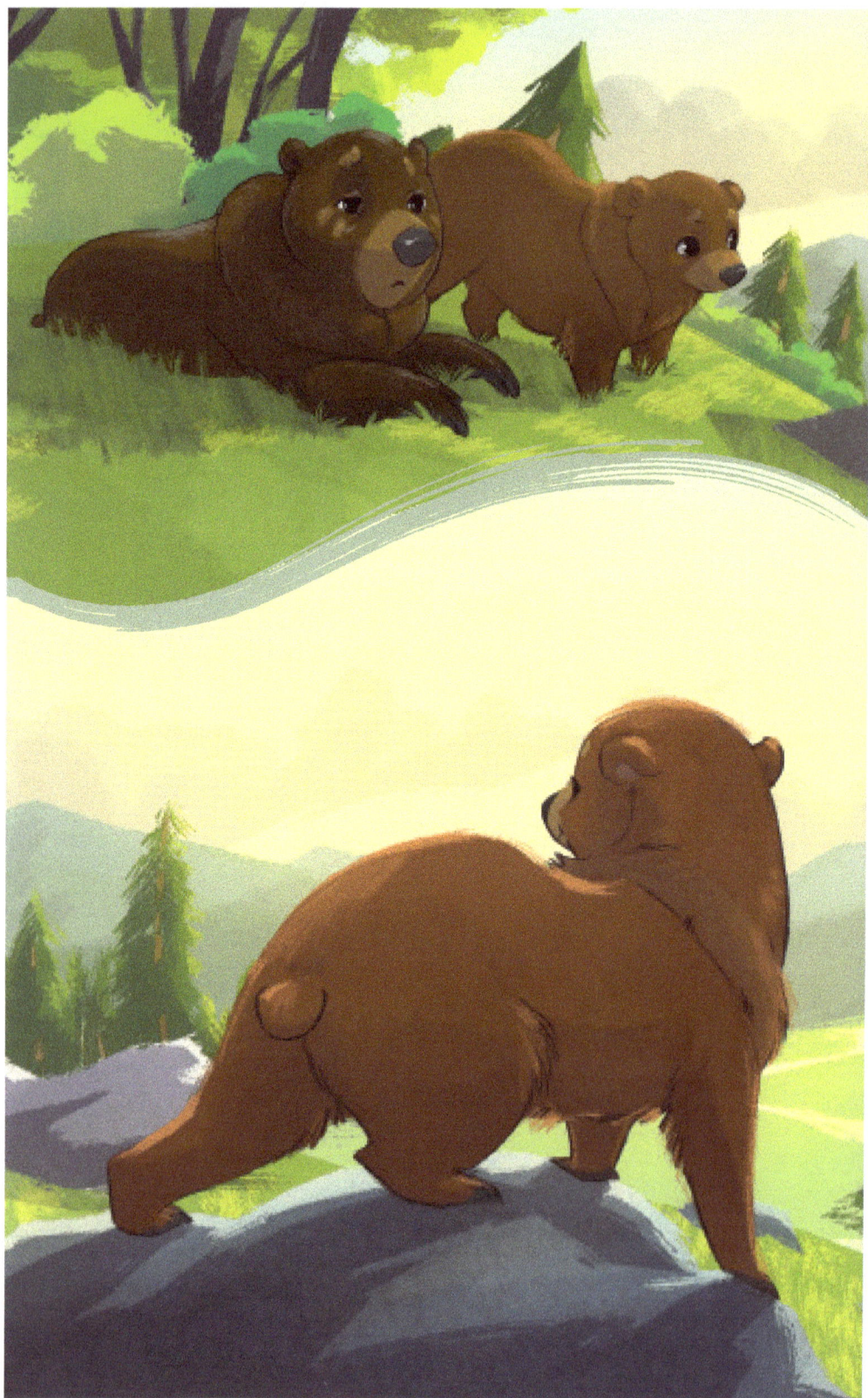

Sister Be<u>a</u>r Moves
to **T<u>e</u>**ton **Na**tion**al** Park

Sister Be<u>a</u>r and her **broth**ers **w<u>a</u>it**ed all day and **in**to the n<u>i</u>ght, **hop**ing their **moth**er would **re**turn. When **morn**ing c<u>a</u>me, **Sis**ter Bear looked to the **moun**tains and then turned to talk to her **broth**ers: "<u>I</u>'m **go**ing to the **moun**tains. **Moth**er said they are **a**m<u>a</u>**zing**, and have a lot of food!"

Big Cub yawned. "We're **hun**gry r<u>i</u>ght now, **Sis**ter Be<u>a</u>r. Y<u>ou</u> can g<u>o</u> to the **moun**tains if y<u>ou</u> want, but **Lit**tle Cub and <u>I</u> are **go**ing to look for food r<u>i</u>ght h<u>e</u>re."

"**O**k<u>ay</u>, then s<u>ee</u> you **some**t<u>i</u>me," said **Sis**ter Be<u>a</u>r. Sh<u>e</u> turned and **head**ed for the **ma**jes**tic** p<u>e</u>aks in the **dis**tance.

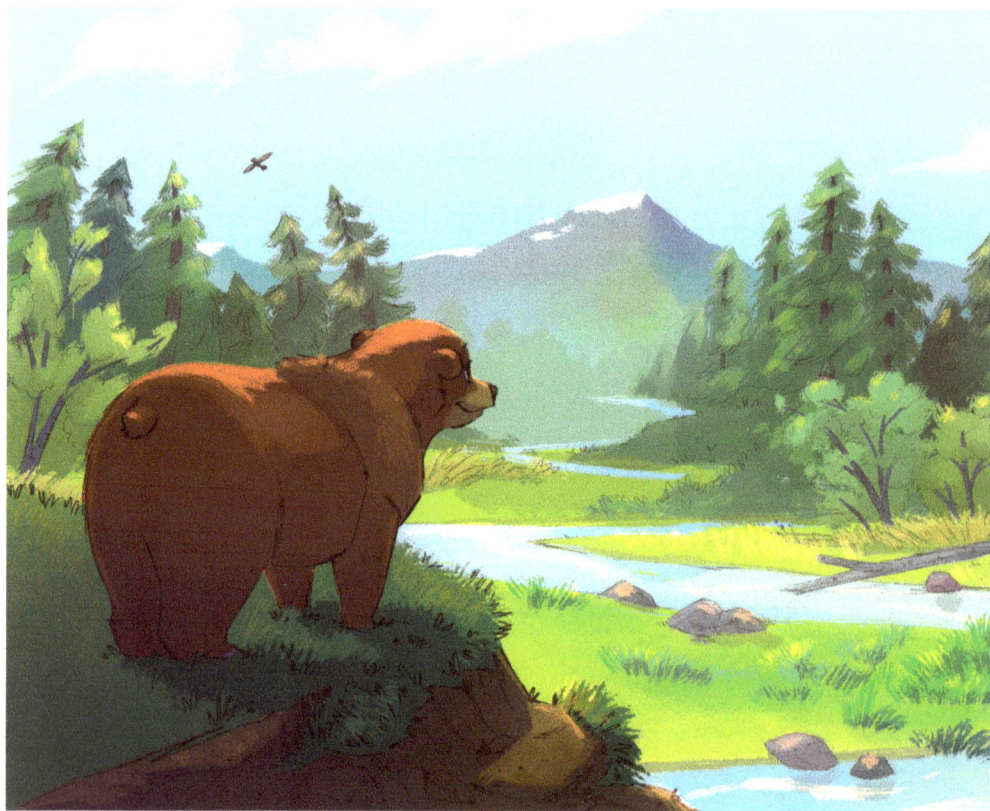

Sister Bear **trav**eled for **man**y days, **liv**ing on **ber**ries, and some voles that she caught in the fields. She walked **a**round large **gey**sers, up and down **moun**tains, **a**long streams, and saw **man**y **animals** as she **trav**eled. Her paws hurt, but she knew she must reach the **moun**tains her **moth**er had told her **a**bout. She climbed to a high peak and looked down over a wide **val**ley with a **crys**tal blue **riv**er **wind**ing through it. There were the **beau**tiful **moun**tains her **moth**er had told her **a**bout. **Sis**ter Bear sniffed the air.

"This will be my **for**ever home!" she said to **her**self. She thought of her **moth**er and wished that she could be there with her. She loved it. There were fish, elk, **huck**le**ber**ries and lots of **veg**etation for her bear beds.

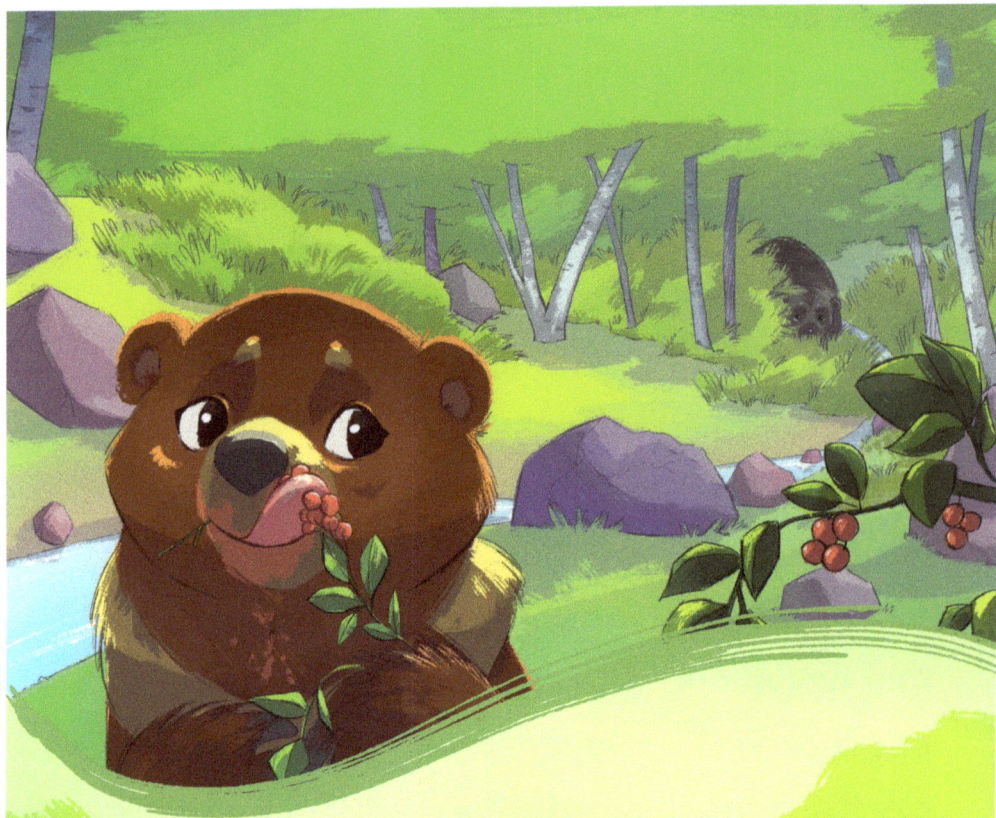

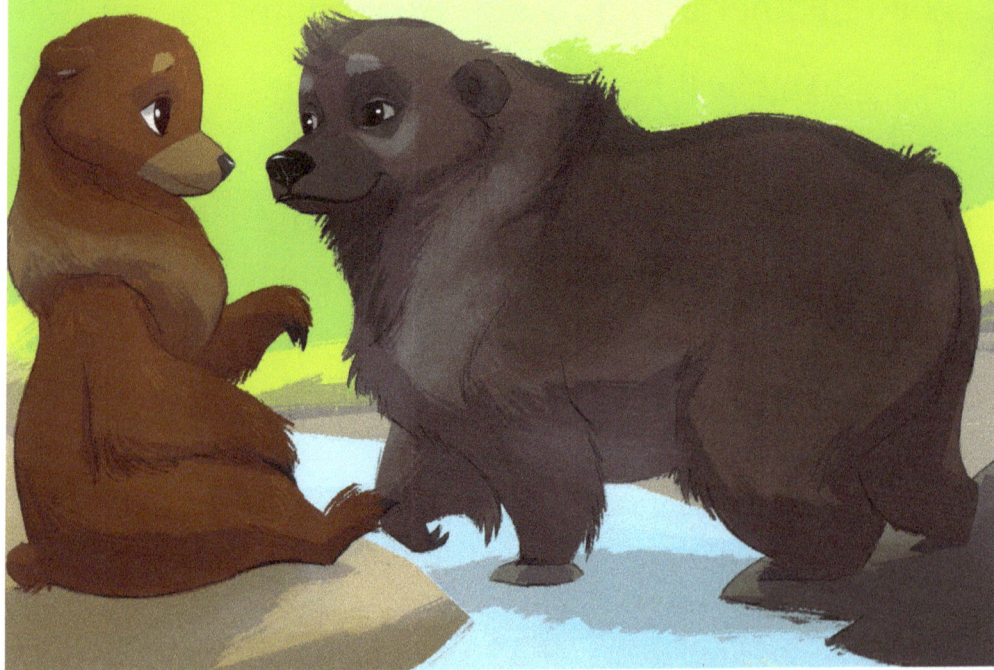

One hot **sum**mer d<u>ay</u>, **Sis**ter Be<u>a</u>r found some **d<u>e</u>licious buffal<u>o</u> ber**ri<u>es</u> and <u>a</u>te **un**til her **muz**zle was **cov**ered in red j<u>ui</u>ce. Sh<u>e</u> went to a str<u>ea</u>m to wash her f<u>a</u>ce. As sh<u>e</u> was **splash**ing **a**bout, **keep**ing her eyes p<u>ee</u>led for a trout or two, sh<u>e</u> heard a noise in the woods.

"Big Cub? **Lit**tle Cub? Is that y<u>ou</u>?" sh<u>e</u> **grunt**ed.

A big m<u>a</u>le <u>**e**</u>merged from the tr<u>ee</u>s.

"Who are y<u>ou</u>?" **Sis**ter Be<u>a</u>r asked, **bat**ting her eyes at him.

The be<u>a</u>r walked up to her. "My n<u>a</u>me is **Br<u>u</u>n<u>o</u>**," h<u>e</u> **r<u>e</u>**plied. H<u>e</u> **b<u>e</u>**gan to lick the **left<u>o</u>ver ber**ry j<u>ui</u>ce from **Sis**ter Be<u>a</u>r's **muz**zle.

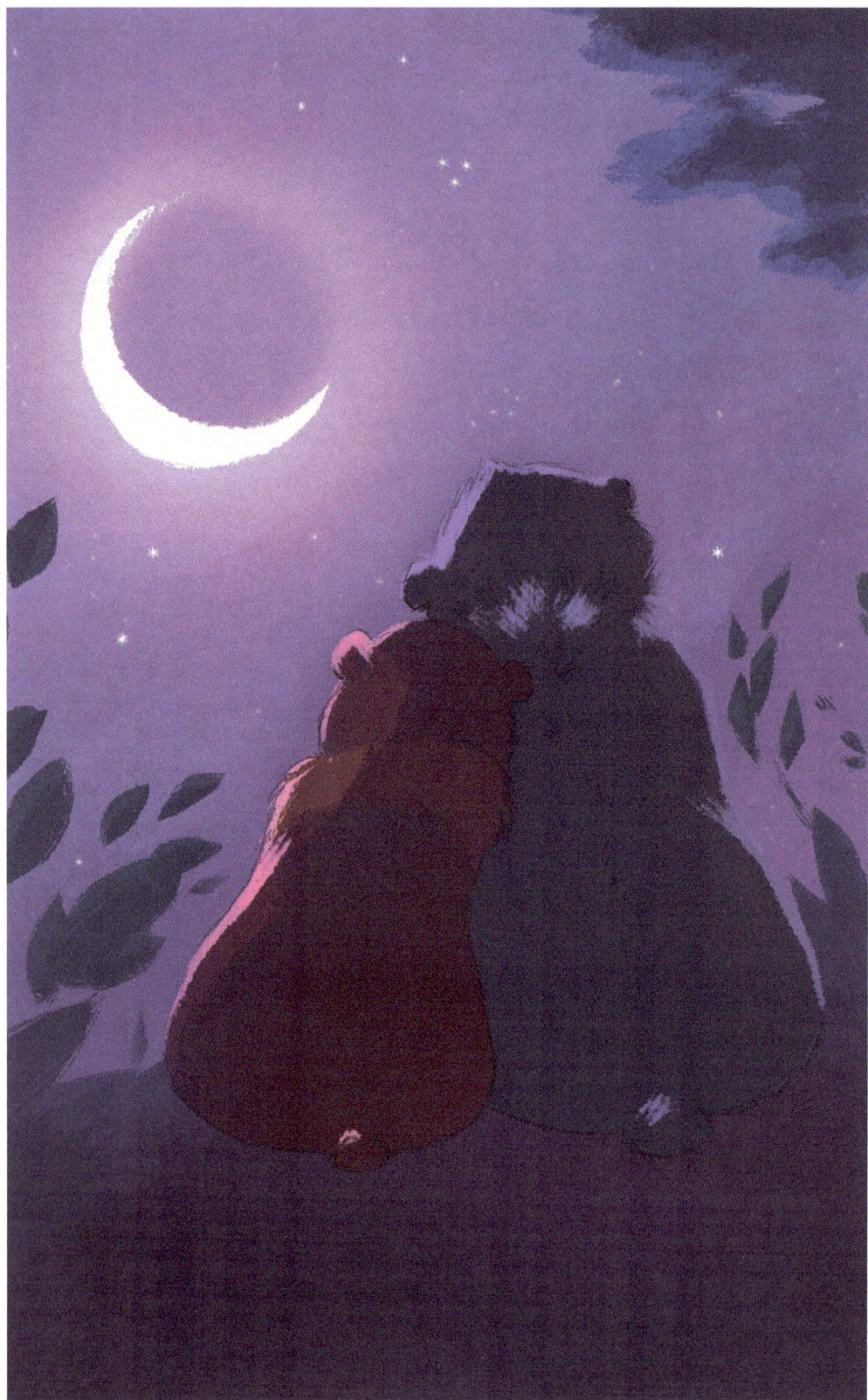

"Want to **bur**row for some voles? I know where there are a lot of them," he said.

"Those are my **fa**vor**ite**!" **ex**claimed **Sis**ter Bear.

The two bears went off to root **a**round for voles. **Sis**ter Bear liked **Bru**no **ver**y much and they **be**came **ver**y close. They stayed **to**gether for a few days, **root**ing **a**round the dirt **dur**ing the day, and **cud**dling **un**der the stars at night as owls **hoot**ed in the trees. One day, **Bru**no roamed off **with**out a word. **Sis**ter Bear was sad, but she **could**n't think **a**bout it. She **need**ed to find food, and **win**ter was **com**ing.

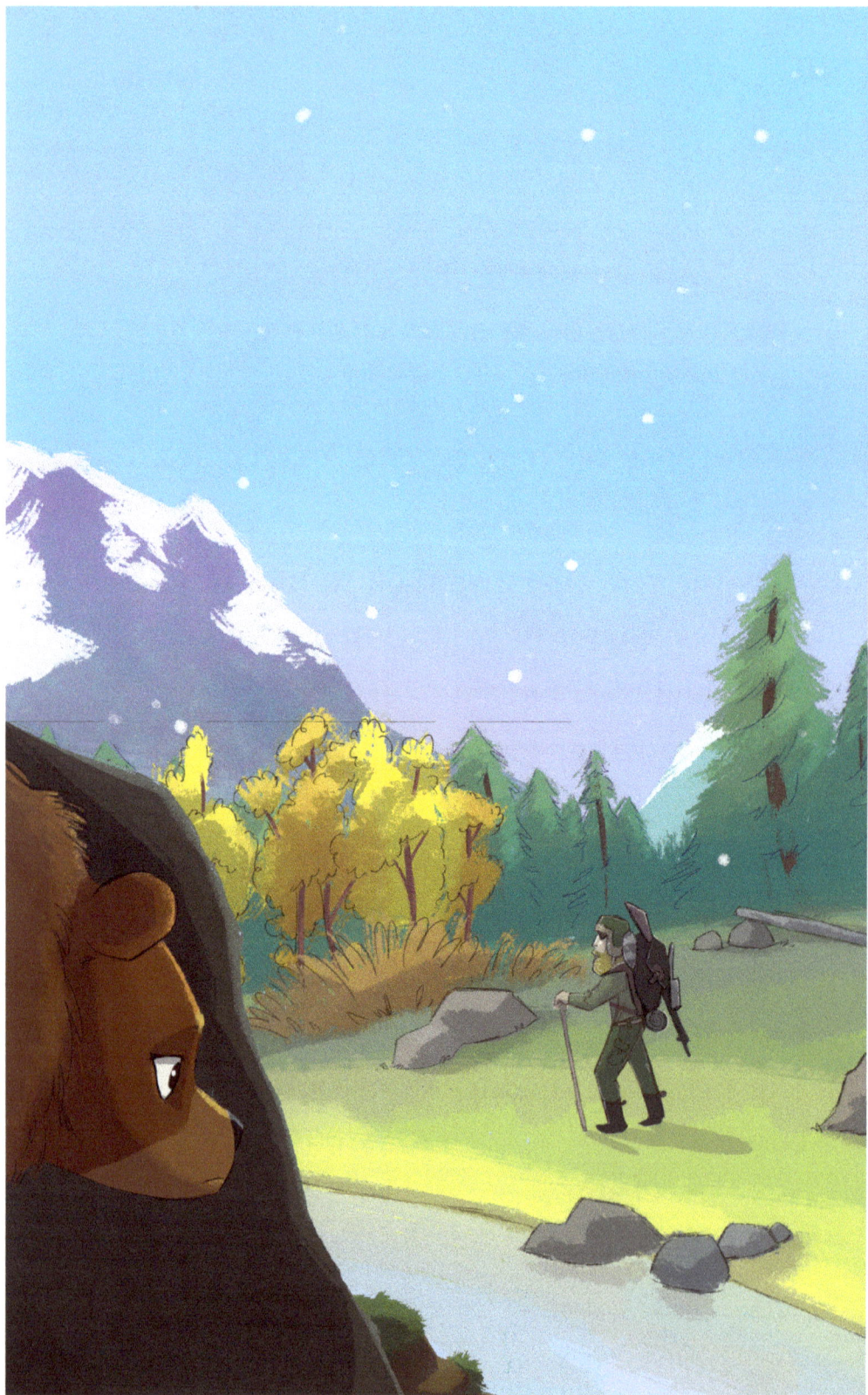

Sister Be<u>a</u>r
Becomes a **Moth**er

Sister Be<u>a</u>r spent the rest of the **sum**mer **find**ing food and <u>ea</u>ting. One d<u>a</u>y, wh<u>i</u>le **for**ag**ing** for food sh<u>e</u> saw a str<u>a</u>nge **an**imal. It walked on two legs and **ca**rri<u>e</u>d some sort of stick that m<u>a</u>de a loud, **boom**ing noise. Sh<u>e</u> **re**mem**bered** her **moth**er **sa**ying **some**thing **a**bout this **animal**; h<u>e</u> was called "man" and that h<u>e</u> **was**n't **al**w<u>a</u>ys **friend**ly and to st<u>a</u>y **a**w<u>a</u>y from him. S<u>o</u>, when sh<u>e</u> saw him, sh<u>e</u> had to st<u>a</u>y **hid**den or move in the **oth**er d<u>i</u>rec**tion**. But as t<u>i</u>me went on and it was **get**ting **cool**er, sh<u>e</u> saw **man**y of th<u>e</u>se men. Sh<u>e</u> would h<u>i</u>de **when**ev**er** sh<u>e</u> saw th<u>e</u>se **cr<u>ea</u>**tures with their **nois**y sticks. The men would shoot their big sticks **kill**ing the elk.

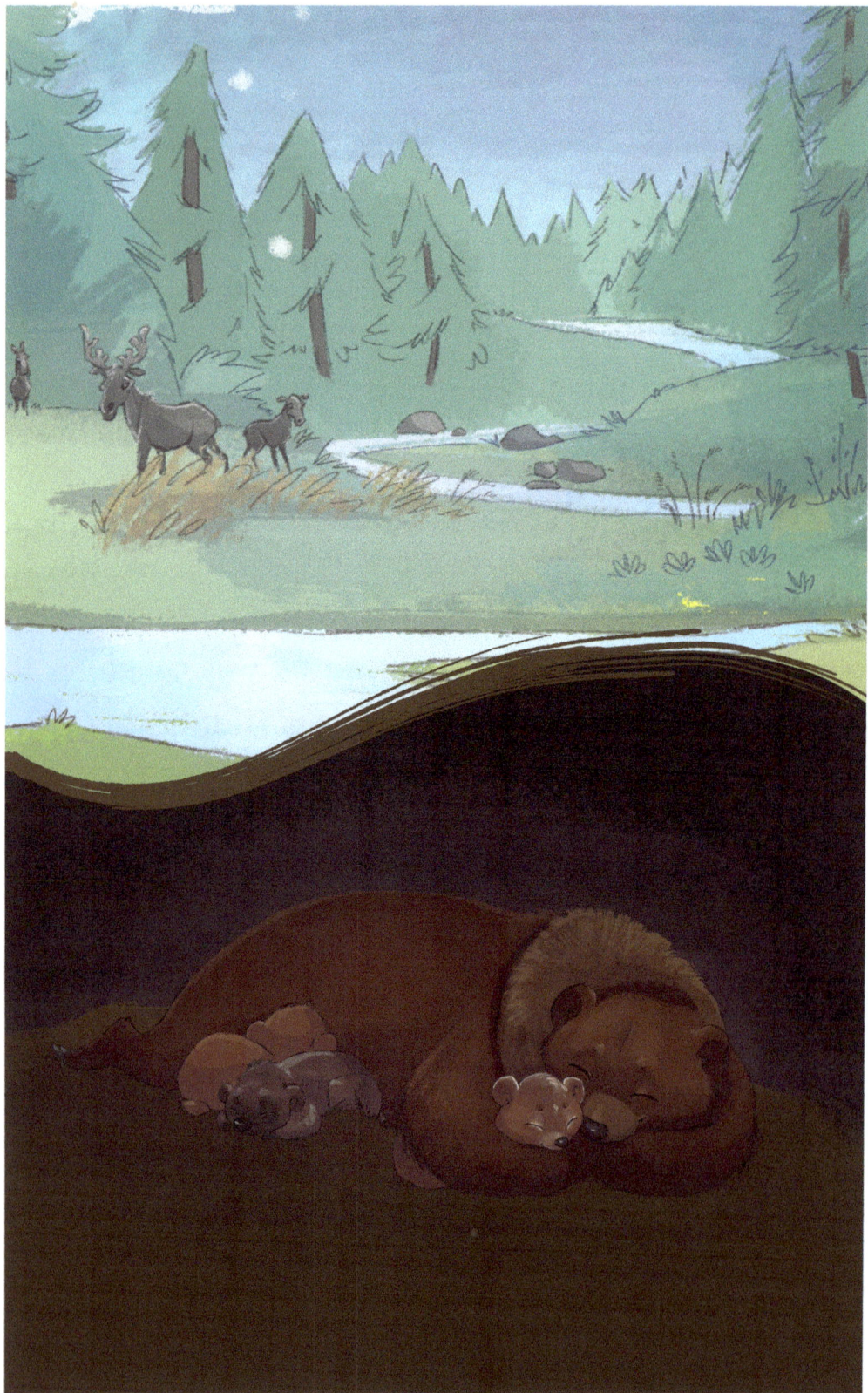

When they left, sh**e** would **qui**etly **wan**der **o**ver and f**ea**st on the **lefto**ver **car**cass. Soon, the sn**ow** **be**gan to fall, and it was t**i**me to g**o** to her den for the **win**ter.

One d**a**y in her **co**zy den, sh**e** g**a**ve birth to thr**ee** c**u**te **lit**tle be**a**r cubs: two **fe**m**a**les and one m**a**le. Sh**e** was **o**ver**joyed** with her new **family**. Sh**e** **nursed** her new **family un**til spring **ar**r**i**ved.

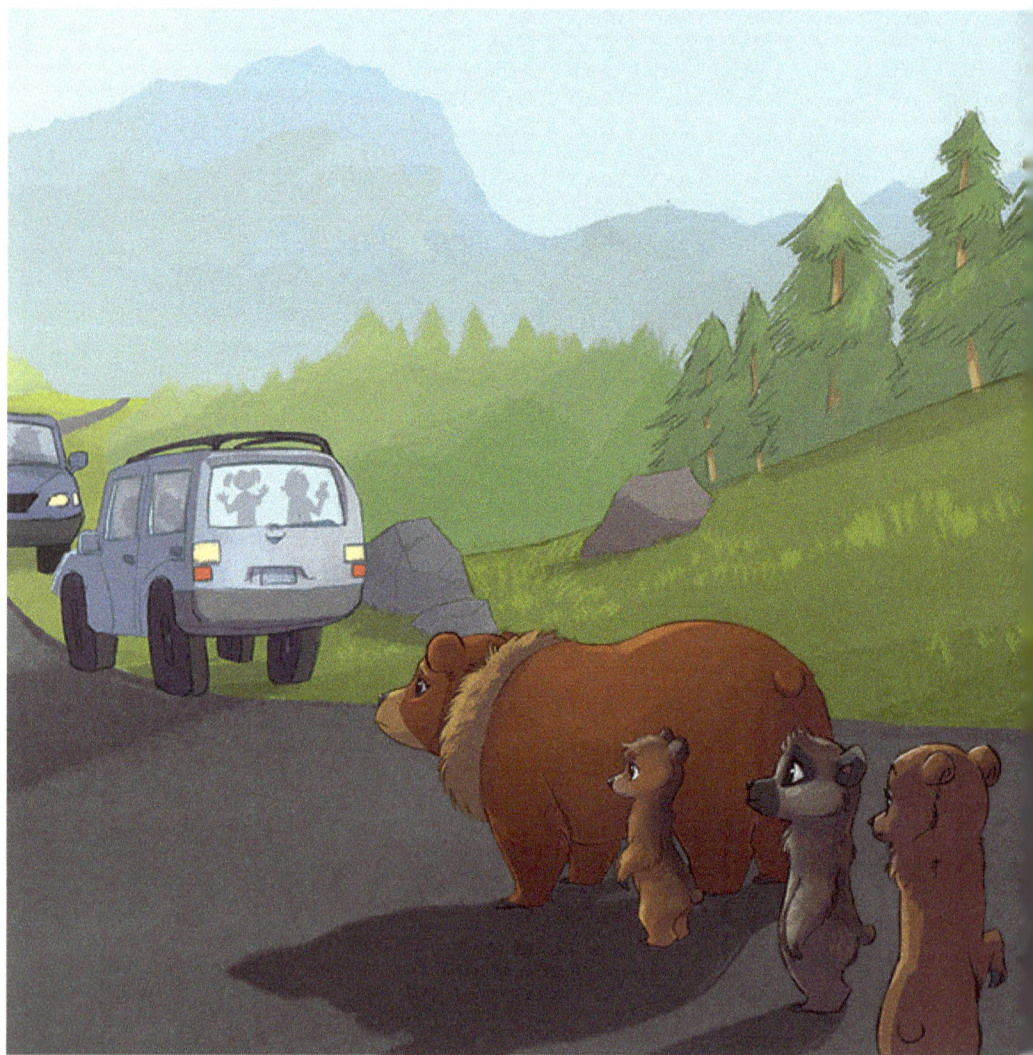

When the sn<u>o</u>w **be**gan to melt and the tr<u>ee</u>s **be**gan to bud, **Sis**ter Bear <u>e</u>merged from her c<u>a</u>ve, with her thr<u>ee</u> **chub**by **lit**tle cubs* **trail**ing **be**hind her. Sh<u>e</u> taught them all the things that her **moth**er had taught her: how to **for**age for **ber**ri<u>e</u>s, to fish, to grub for moths, and to st<u>ea</u>l **cach**es of **White**bark p<u>i</u>ne nuts from **squir**rels. Sh<u>e</u> **al**s<u>o</u> taught them to **a**void man. **Some**times, as they r<u>o</u>amed thr<u>ou</u>gh their h<u>o</u>me in the **na**tion**al** park, they would s<u>ee</u> l<u>i</u>nes of cars on the r<u>o</u>ads filled with **hu**mans.

The **hu**mans would often have **cam**er**as** or cell ph<u>o</u>nes in their hands, **ta**k**ing** **ph<u>o</u>**tos of the Be<u>a</u>r **fam**ily as they passed by. This **hap**pened **fre**quent**ly**, and the **pe<u>o</u>**ple s<u>ee</u>med **ver**y **hap**py to s<u>ee</u> them. Soon, they got <u>u</u>sed to the **pe<u>o</u>**ple.

* The **ba**by be<u>a</u>rs were **la**ter **giv**en **num**bers by the **Na**tion**al** Park **Ser**vice and **re**ferred to as #610, #615, and #549.

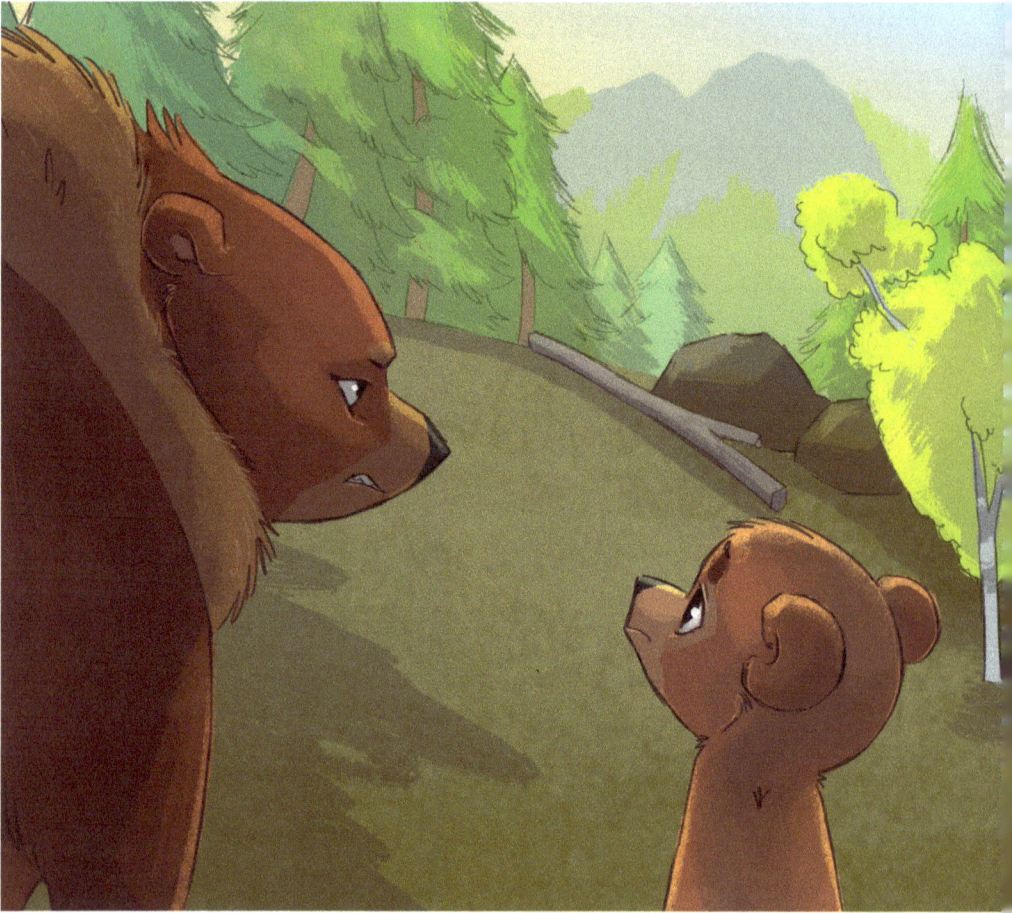

The **Im**pacts of Man

Sometimes, **Sis**ter Bear would try to cross the road where men were **driv**ing their cars. This made her **nerv**ous, but she taught her cubs to move **quick**ly **a**way from them and how to **a**void the cars. Last year, she had a **ba**by cub named Snowy – but **sad**ly **Snow**y was hit by a car. It had made her **very** sad, but she learned a lot **a**bout fast **traveling vehicles**. **Be**cause of this, she taught her cubs to look both ways **be**fore **cross**ing the road. Most of the time they **lis**tened if they weren't **dis**tract**ed play**ing with each **oth**er.

One **sun**ny spring day, **Sis**ter Bear and her cubs were **fin**ish**ing** off a **tast**y moose. She heard a noise and stood up on her back legs, **sniff**ing the air. A man **wear**ing a hat **sud**den**ly** came **up**on them. He stopped and stared at them.

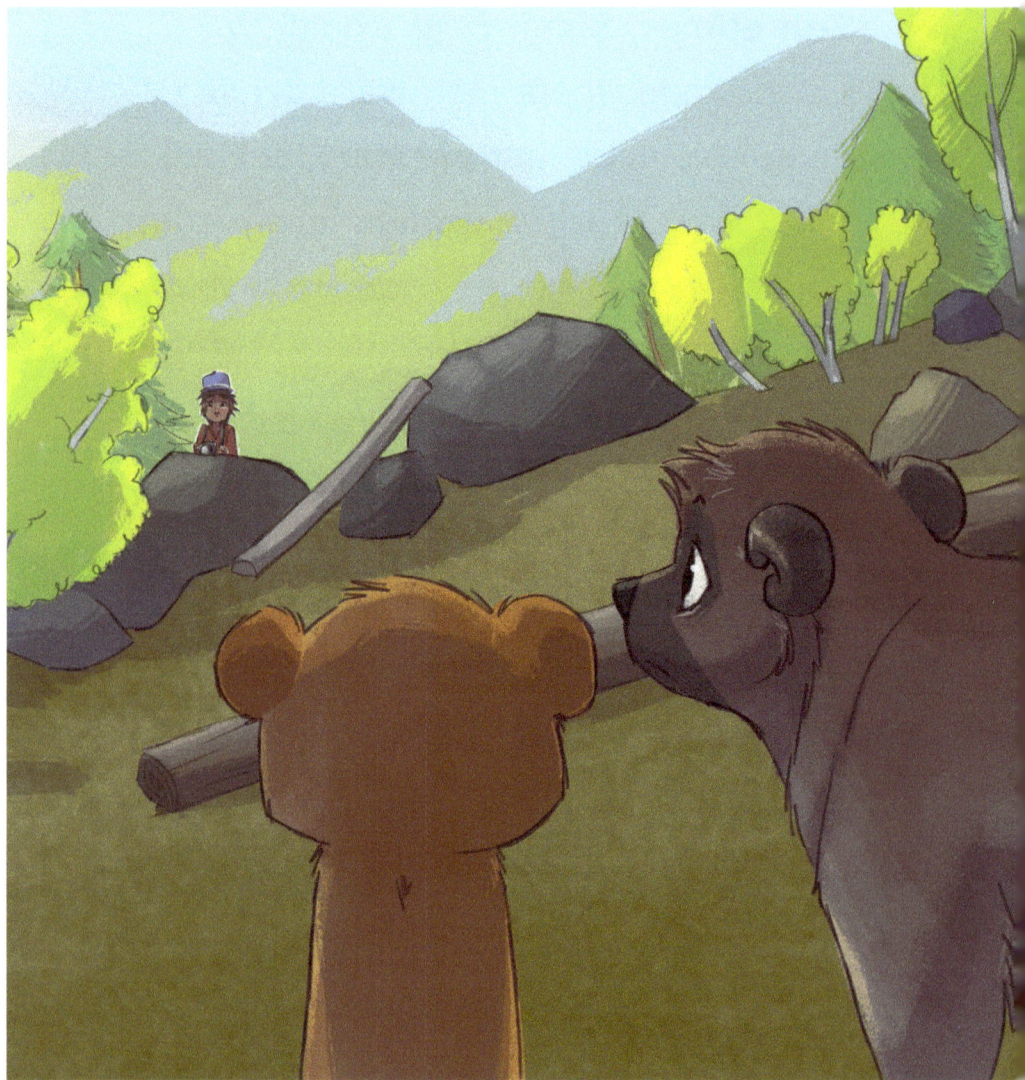

"**Mom**ma!" the **lit**tle **fe**male cub cr<u>i</u>ed.
"Will h<u>e</u> t<u>a</u>ke our food?"

Sister Be<u>a</u>r let out a **deaf**en**ing** roar.
"N<u>o</u>, my **lit**tle one! H<u>e</u> w<u>o</u>n't!"

Sister Be<u>a</u>r ran **to**wards the man and
knocked him to the ground. His hat flew off
and h<u>e</u> **be**gan to yell. Sh<u>e</u> then sat down on
top of him and **start**ed to b<u>i</u>te his head. Her
cubs c<u>a</u>me **run**ning, **call**ing out to her.

"**Mom**ma! Yo<u>u</u> said w<u>e</u> were to l<u>ea</u>ve man
a<u>lo</u>ne!" they cr<u>i</u>ed.

Sister Be<u>a</u>r growled once more and then
got up, **let**ting the man g<u>o</u> fr<u>ee</u>. H<u>e</u> grabbed
his hat and ran **a**w<u>ay</u> **to**wards the woods.

"You're r<u>i</u>ght, **chil**dren. <u>I</u>'m sure moose
t<u>a</u>stes much **bet**ter, **an**yw<u>ay</u>!"

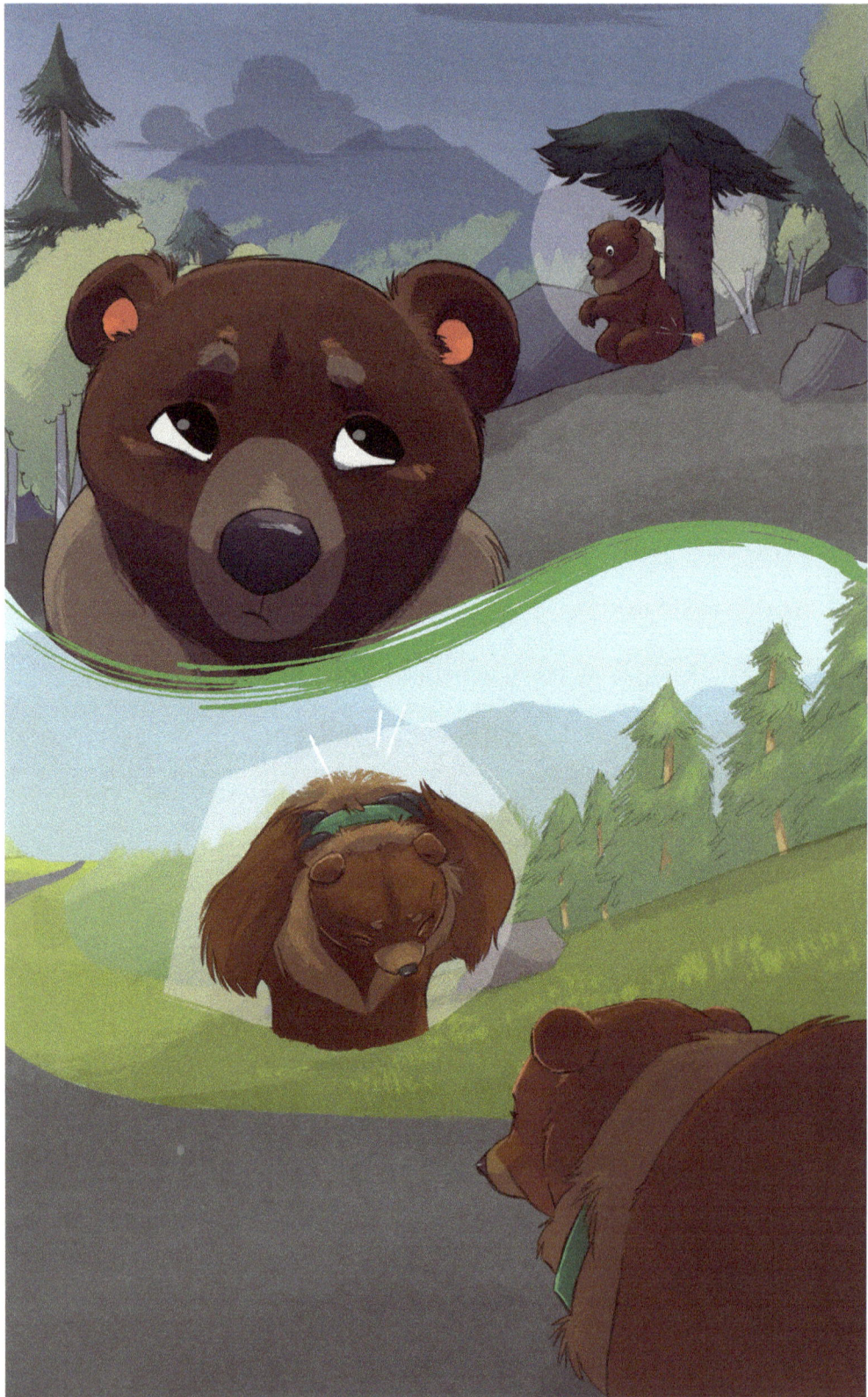

Chapter 5

Sister Be<u>a</u>r **Be**comes **Griz**zly 399

Later that **sum**mer, as storm clouds blew in from the west, **Sis**ter Be<u>a</u>r was **scratch**ing her rump **a**gainst a p<u>i</u>ne tr<u>ee</u>. **Sud**den**ly**, sh<u>e</u> felt a sharp sting and sh<u>e</u> **be**gan to f<u>ee</u>l **ver**y **sl<u>ee</u>p**y...When sh<u>e</u> **a**w<u>o</u>ke, sh<u>e</u> had a str<u>a</u>nge ring **a**round her thick, **fur**ry neck and **plas**tic things on her <u>e</u>ars*. **Sis**ter Be<u>a</u>r went **cr<u>a</u>zy try**ing to get the **col**lar off. Sh<u>e</u> would rub it **a**gainst logs, scratch at it with her h<u>u</u>ge claws, and sh<u>e</u> <u>e</u>ven let her cubs chew on it. Sh<u>e</u> worked **ver**y hard to **re**move it and with one big yank, sh<u>e</u> got the **col**lar off.

But, in n<u>o</u> time, the s<u>a</u>me thing **hap**pened: sh<u>e</u> went to sl<u>ee</u>p and w<u>o</u>ke up **wea**ring **an**oth**er col**lar! **Pe<u>o</u>**ple in gr<u>ee</u>n <u>u</u>ni**forms** were **al**w<u>a</u>ys **watch**ing her. But sh<u>e</u> was an **es**c<u>a</u>pe **art**ist and would **re**move the **col**lar **eve**ry t<u>i</u>me!

* The **Nati<u>o</u>nal** Park **Ser**vice assigned her the **num**ber 399, which is how sh<u>e</u> got her n<u>a</u>me.

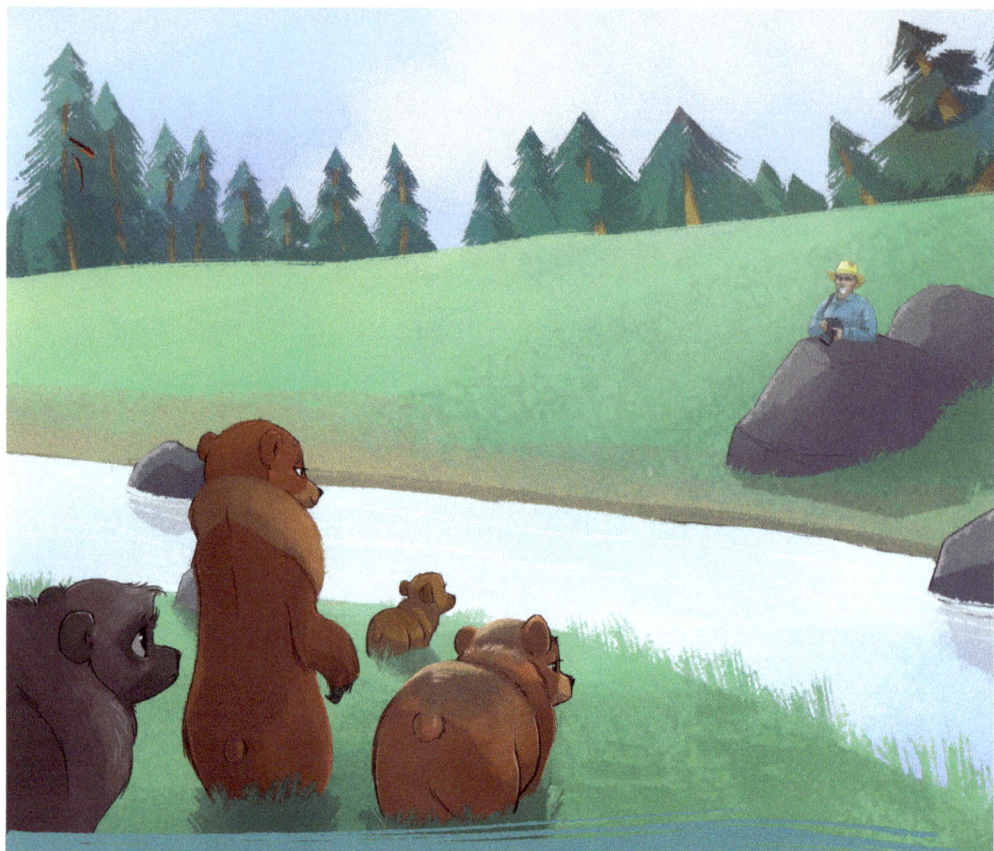

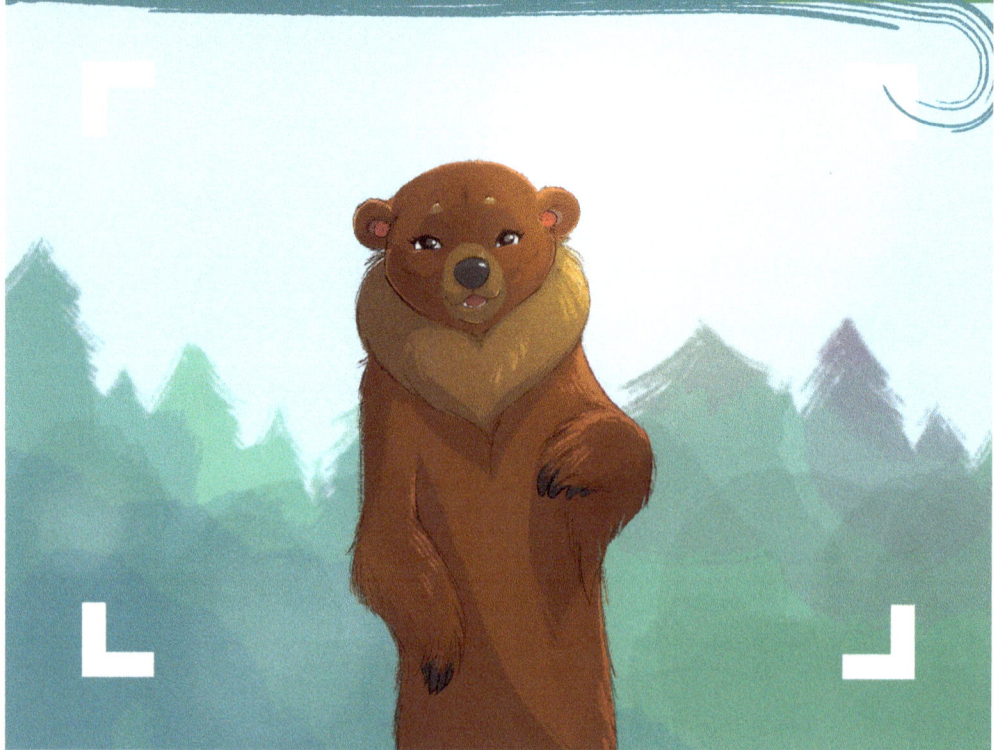

Grizzly 399 M<u>ee</u>ts
a **F<u>a</u>**mous **Ph<u>o</u>**tog**ra**pher

There was **als<u>o</u> an**oth**er** man who **fol**l<u>o</u>wed her **a**round the **moun**tains. H<u>e</u> didn't s<u>ee</u>m **threat**en**ing**—**in**stead of a stick, h<u>e</u> had this thing on a strap **a**round his neck that went click-click. H<u>e</u> **nev**er c<u>a</u>me cl<u>o</u>se to her or her cubs.

Sister Be<u>a</u>r, now kn<u>o</u>wn as **Gri**zzly 399, got <u>u</u>sed to the man **hang**ing **a**round with his **lit**tle box. **Some**times, sh<u>e</u> would stand up and p<u>o</u>se for him, **sh<u>o</u>w**ing her h<u>u</u>ge be<u>a</u>r t<u>ee</u>th in a big be<u>a</u>r sm<u>i</u>le!

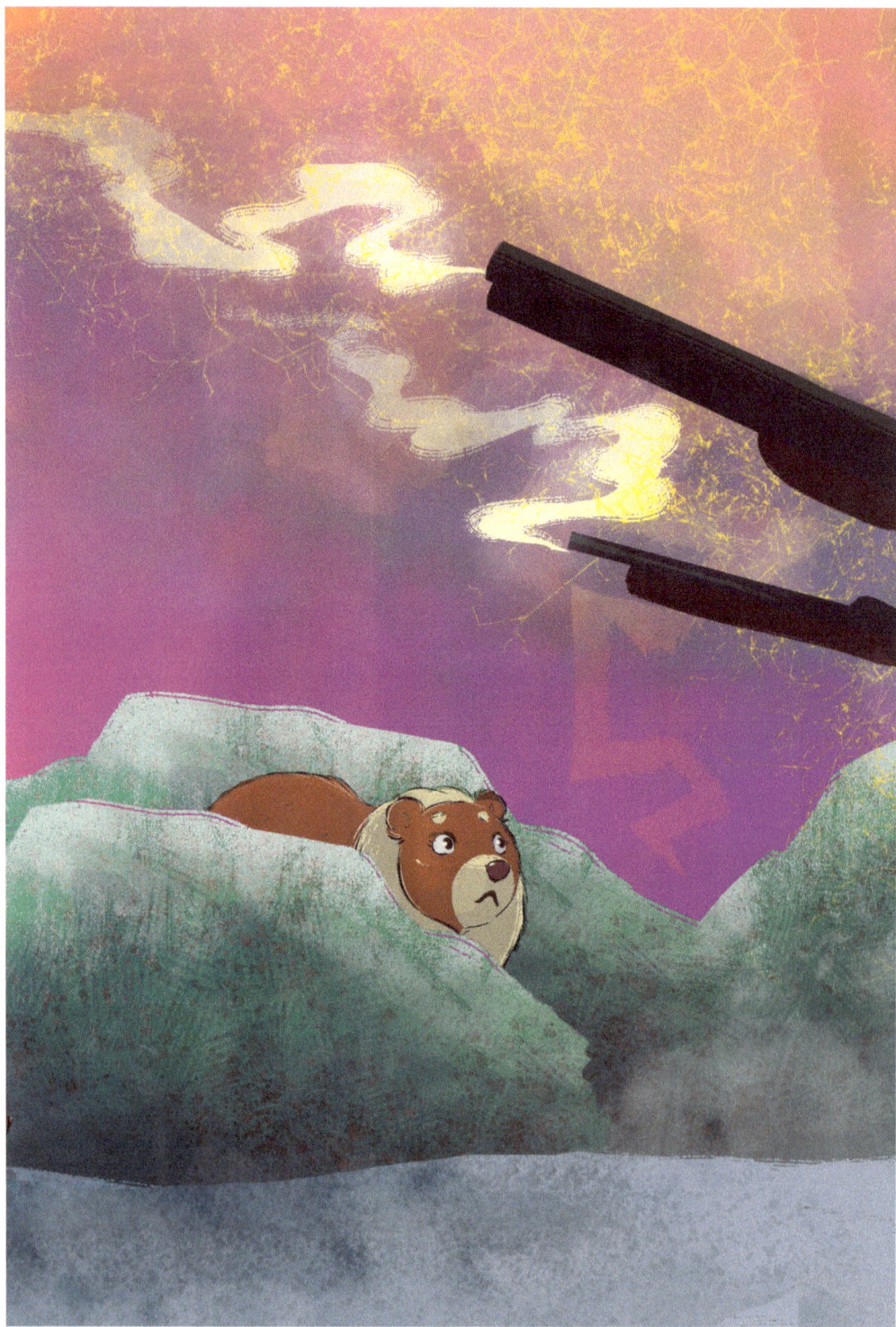

As fall **con**tin**ued**, she taught her **ba**bies **a**bout the **hunt**ers and how to **a**void them. Once, they walked close by a line of men with the big sticks. She told her **ba**bies, "Keep **qui**et and stay **a**way from them. The men **nev**er saw them. That year, **Griz**zly 399 and her cubs stayed up late **in**to the **win**ter months so they could eat more **left**overs left by the **hunt**ers.

When the cubs third spring **ar**rived, **Griz**zly 399 told them, "Cubs, it is time for you to go on your own! My **moth**er did this to me and my **broth**ers. Now it's time for you to find your way and one day have your own **fam**ilies."

Saying this, she walked **a**way from her **be**wil**dered** cubs, **leav**ing them al**o**ne.

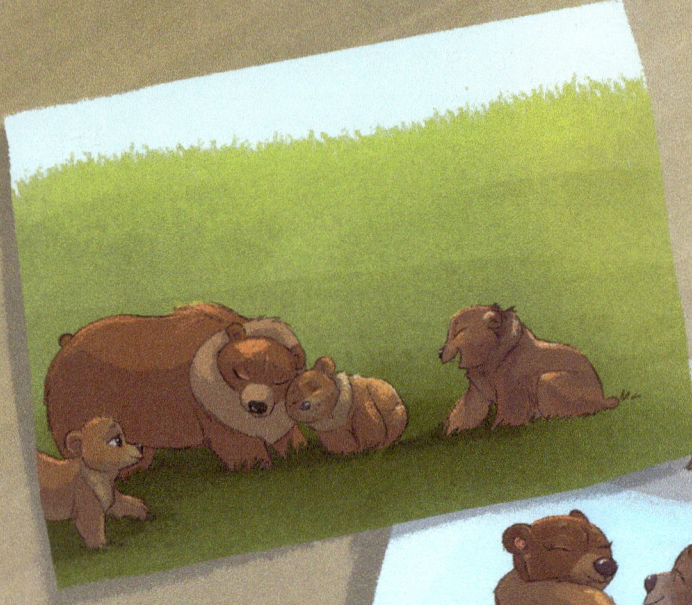

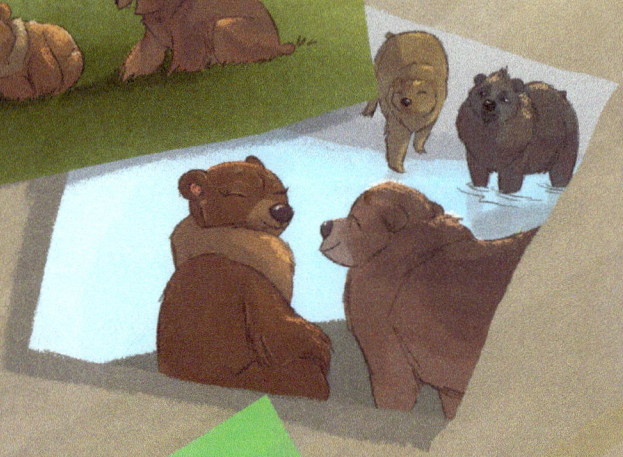

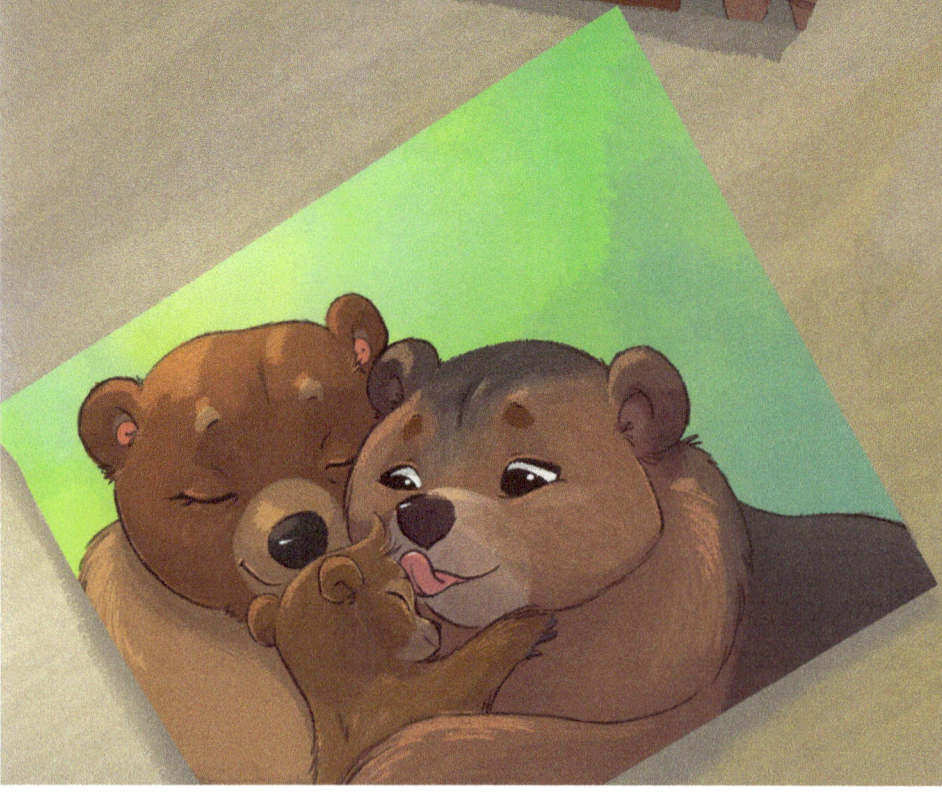

Grizzly 399 the
Best **Moth**er Bear of All Time

Seasons passed and **Sis**ter Bear had more cubs. In turn, her cubs had **ba**bies as well. In the **spring**time, they would meet up along the streams and in the **val**leys.

Another year went by, and **Griz**zly 399 had just come out of her den with three more **ba**by cubs. Out of the **cor**ner of her eye, she saw her **daugh**ter **Griz**zly 610 **com**ing **to**wards her with two **ba**by cubs **be**hind her. She thought, Oh my **ba**by girl had cubs! She told her cubs, "Kids, we can play and eat with them, but not for too long!"

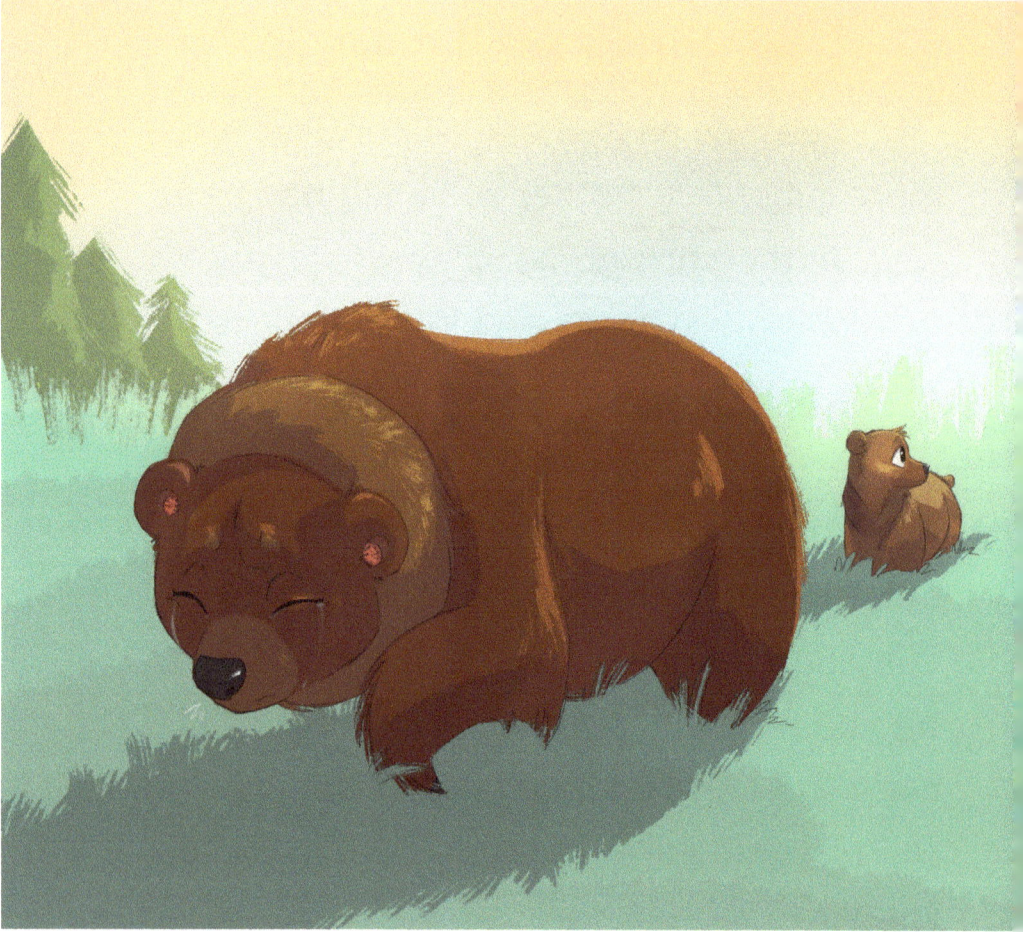

Sister Bear **no**ticed that her **daugh**ter **Griz**zly 610, her **first**born, had **tak**en a **lik**ing to one of her **young**est boy cubs and he was **close**ly fol**low**ing her.

Grizzly 399 looked at **Griz**zly 610 and said, "You can raise him if you want – he wants to be with you!"

Grizzly 610 **nod**ded and went off **in**to the **moun**tains with the **lit**tle cub **fol**low**ing** close **be**hind. **Griz**zly 610 had now **be**come his **a**dopt**ed moth**er.

One **chil**ly **au**tumn day, **Griz**zly 399 was **search**ing for her two young cubs. They had **wan**dered off, **for**ag**ing** for **ber**ries. This set of cubs were full of **mis**chief and **al**ways liked to hide in the thick, dark pines.

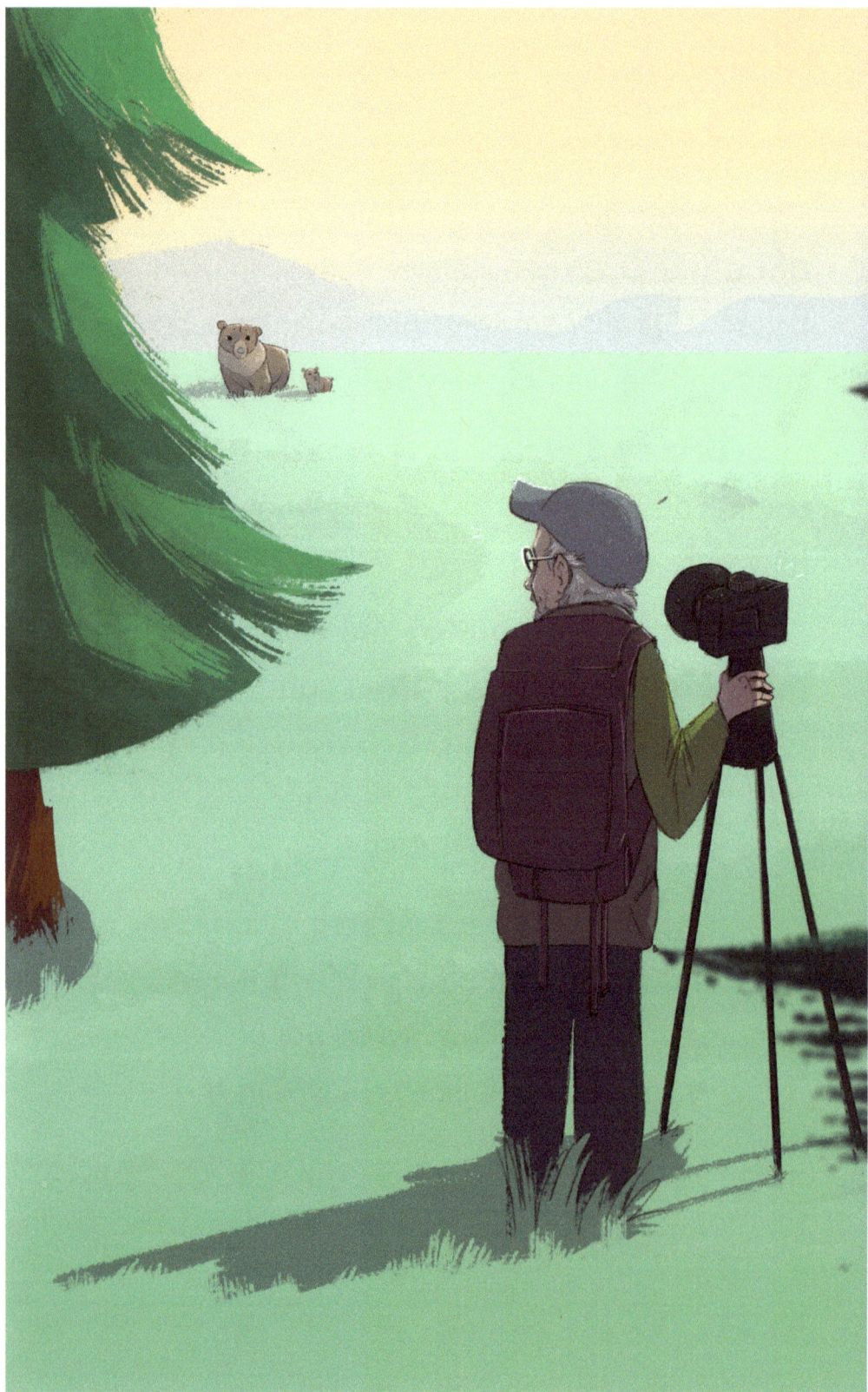

Grizzly 399 stood up on her h<u>i</u>nd legs and took some d<u>ee</u>p breaths, **try**ing to catch her cubs' scent in the wind. Sh<u>e</u> **frantical**ly looked for her **lit**tle ones but **could**n't find them **any**where. Sh<u>e</u> sat down in the **mid**dle of a **gold**en **mead**<u>o</u>w and **be**gan to cry.

A **m**<u>o</u>ment **lat**er, sh<u>e</u> saw the **friend**ly man. Click-click went the thing **a**round his neck. Sh<u>e</u> knew his smell **be**cause sh<u>e</u> saw him **of**ten. Sh<u>e</u> was not **a**fr<u>ai</u>d of him – for in a sense sh<u>e</u> felt h<u>e</u> c<u>a</u>red **a**bout her. The man **spot**ted her and **nod**ded **to**ward some tr<u>ee</u>s. **Griz**zly 399 looked **to**ward the p<u>i</u>nes and saw her cubs **run**ning **to**wards her. Sh<u>e</u> glanced at the man and g<u>a</u>ve one **fi**nal roar to s<u>ay</u>, "Thank yo<u>u</u>."

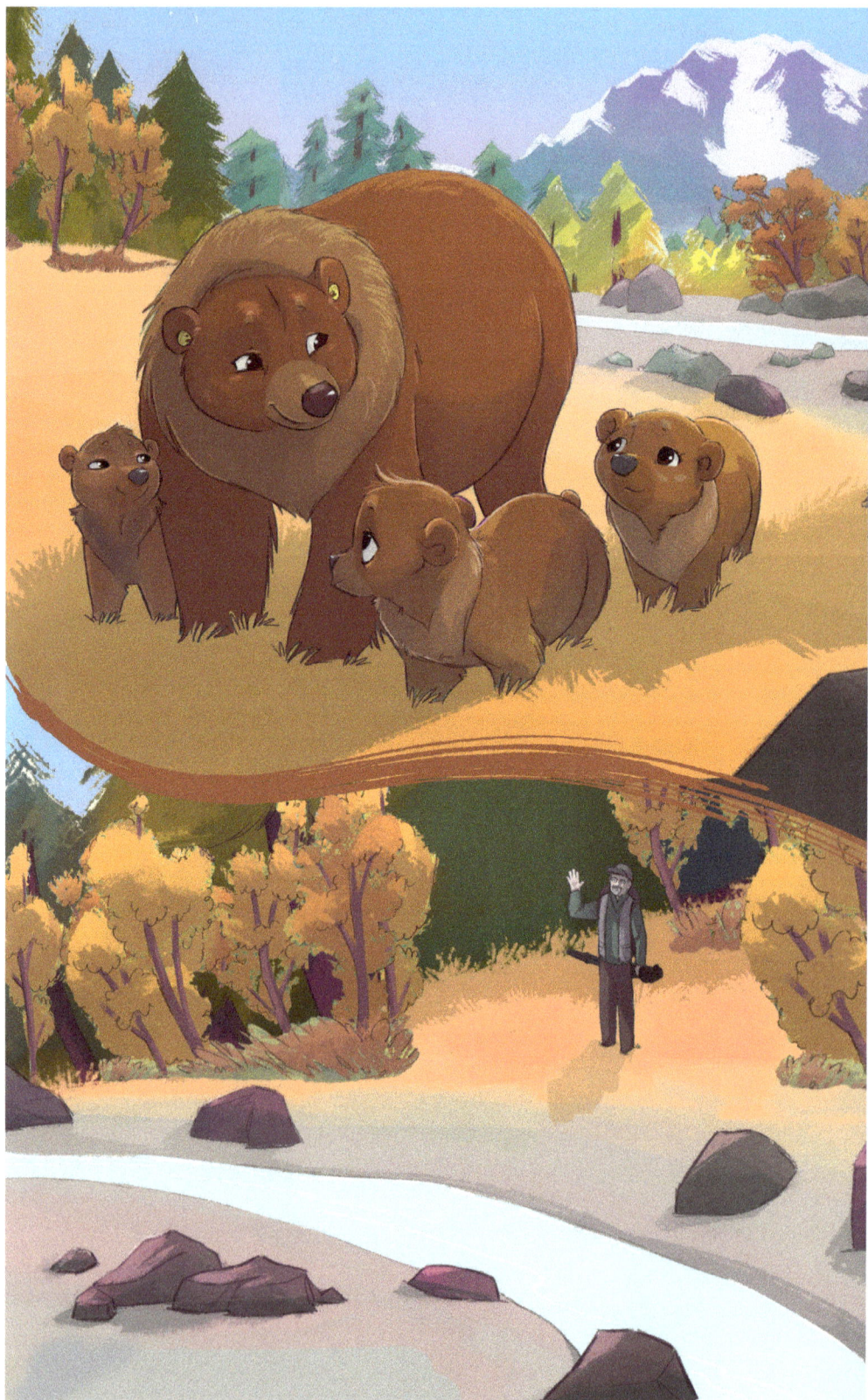

Winter was **com**ing and it was time to find a den to **hi**ber**nate** in. **Griz**zly 399 gazed at the man one last time **be**fore **head**ing **to**ward the high peaks. She caught his scent on the breeze as he raised his arm and waved to her. She knew she would see him **a**gain, when the spring **flow**ers bloomed.

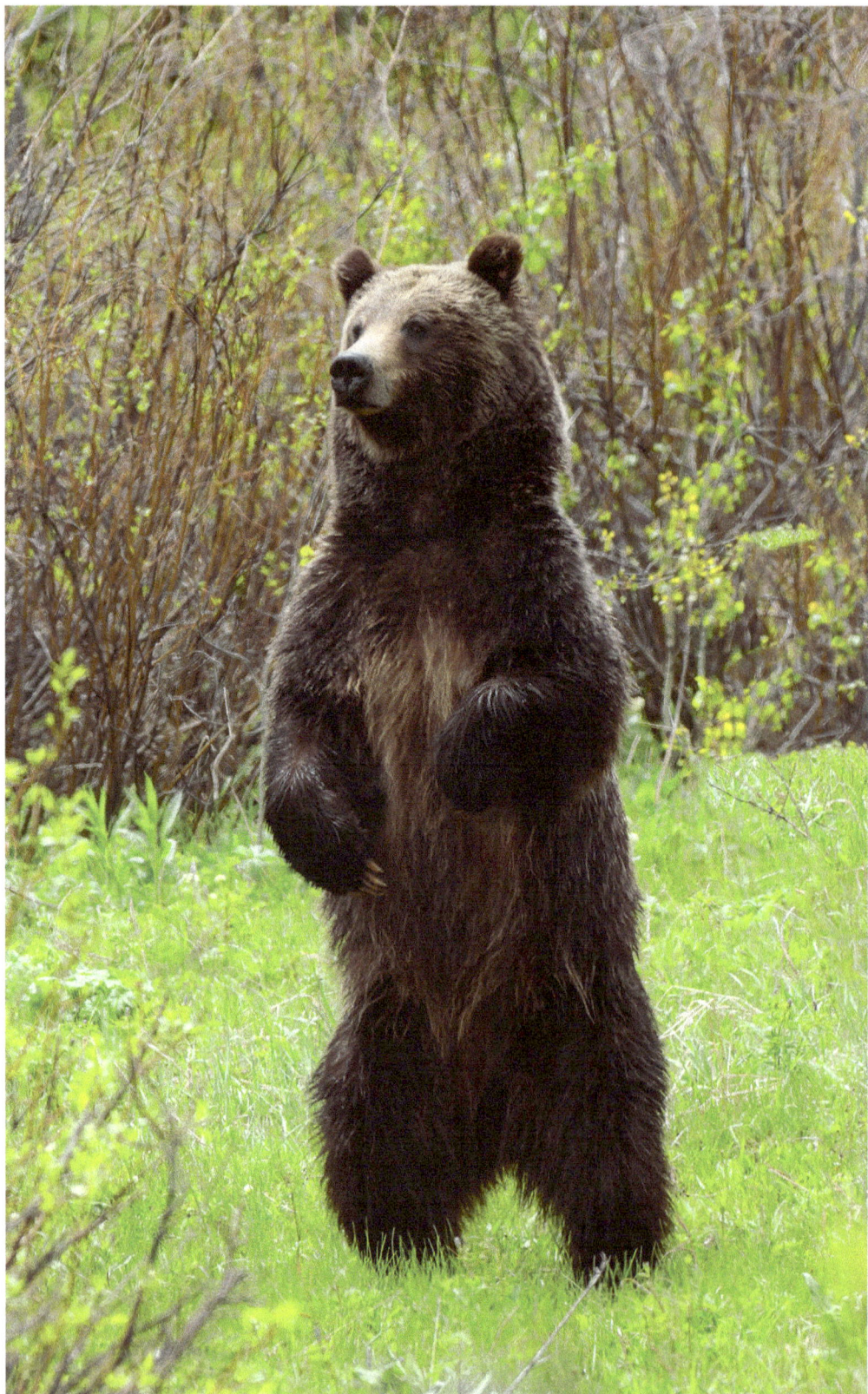

Meet the **Re**al **Griz**zly 399

Grizzly 399 is a **mag**nificent **fe**male grizzly bear **liv**ing in Grand **Te**ton **Na**tional Park and its **sur**round**ings**.

She was born in the **win**ter of 1996 in the **Yel**low**stone** - **Te**ton **E**cosystem.

In 2006, she was **spot**ted in **north**ern Grand **Te**ton **Na**tional Park with three cubs (as told in this **stor**y). **O**ver the next 18 years, she gave birth to a **to**tal of 22 cubs with **man**y of her **off**spring **also** hav**ing** their own cubs.

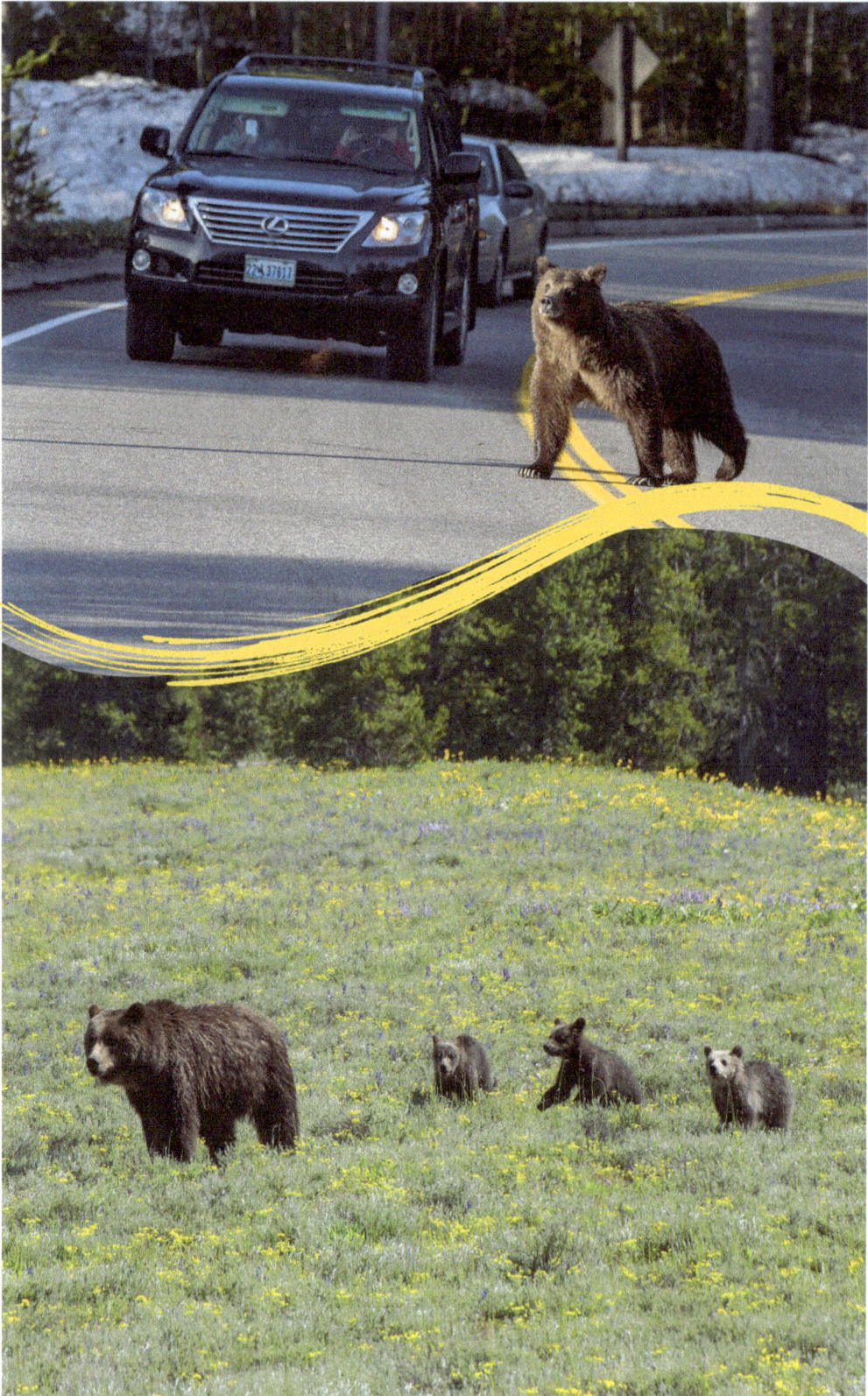

Grizzly 399 gained **popularity** due to her **frequent appearances** along the **road**sides of **Te**ton **National** Park. She chose these **locations** to **pro**tect her young from male bears, who **most**ly stayed in the **back**country.

News spread among **tour**ists and **pho**togra**phers that **Griz**zly 399 and her cubs were **easily visible** from the **road**side. As a **re**sult, **mil**lions of **tour**ists flocked to the park to see this **beau**tiful **i**con**ic mother** bear and her cubs.

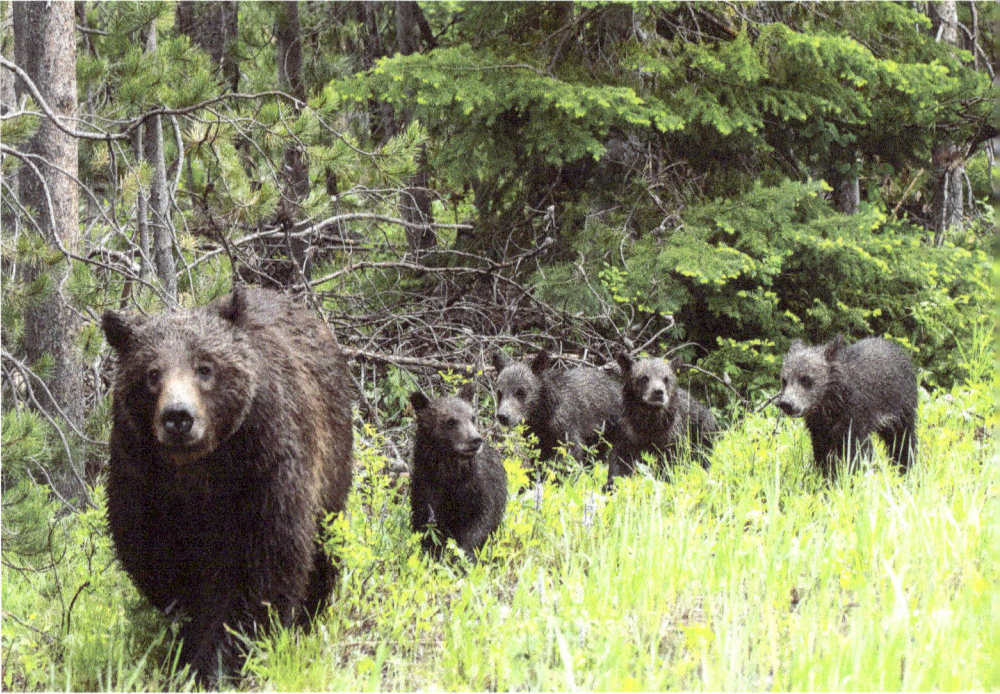

In the Spring of 2020, **Griz**zly 399 **sur**prised the world by **giv**ing birth to four **a**dorable cubs. At the time of their birth, she was 24 years old, which is **con**sid**ered** quite old for a **griz**zly bear to have **ba**bies.

Giving birth to these four cubs **so**lid**if**ied her **sta**tus as the most **fa**mous **griz**zly bear of all time!

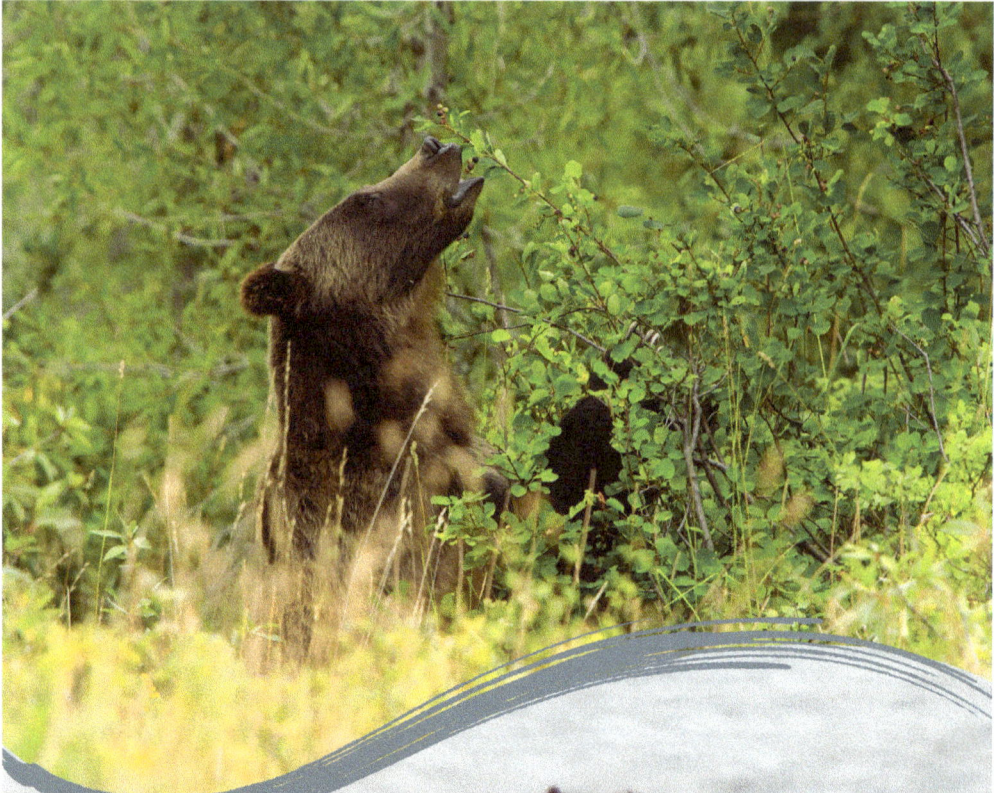

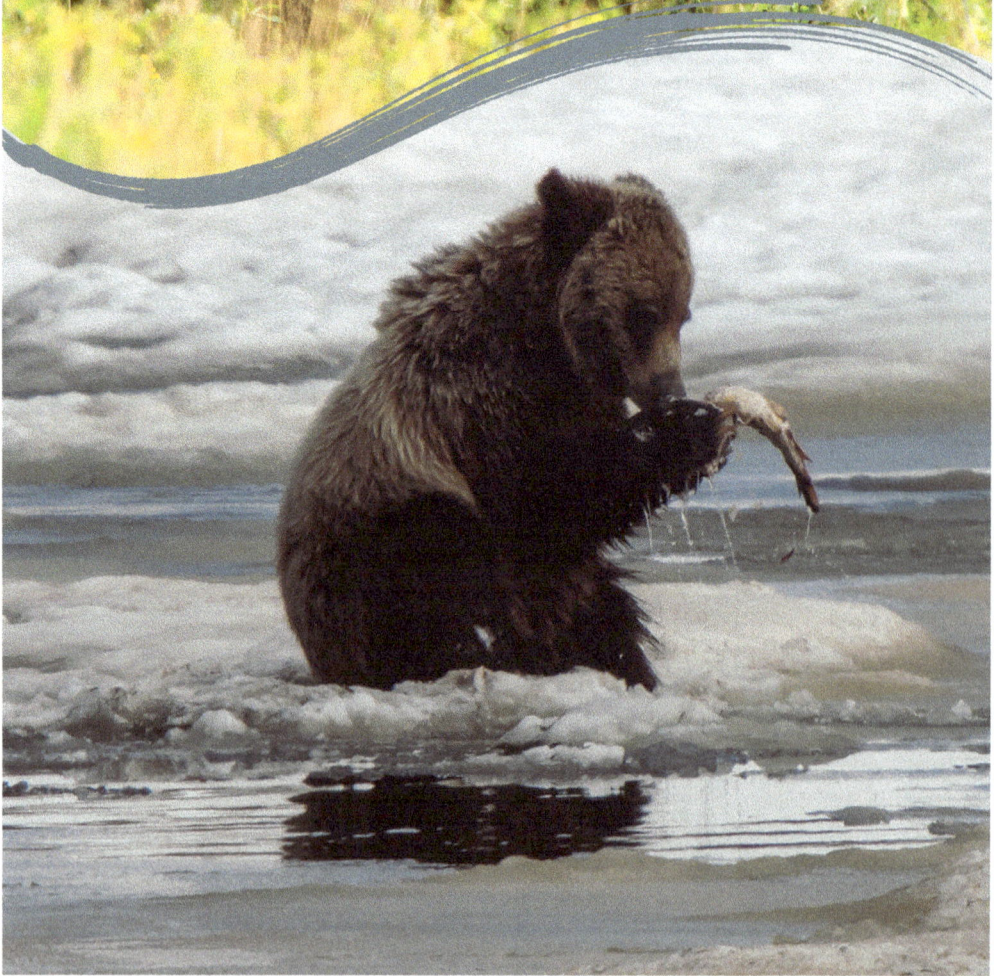

Grizzly 399 has taught her cubs to:

- Look b<u>o</u>th w<u>a</u>ys when **cross**ing the r<u>o</u>ad.
- F<u>i</u>nd food l<u>i</u>ke **wh<u>i</u>te**bark p<u>i</u>ne s<u>ee</u>ds, **ber**ri<u>e</u>s, bugs, and dead **an**i**mals**.
- Catch fish <u>e</u>ven in <u>i</u>cy **wa**ters.
- **Scav**enge for elk guts **dur**ing the
- s<u>ea</u>sonal elk hunt in **Te**ton **Na**tional park.
- Hunt elk calves at **Wi**ll<u>o</u>w Flats and **oth**er **mead**<u>o</u>ws.

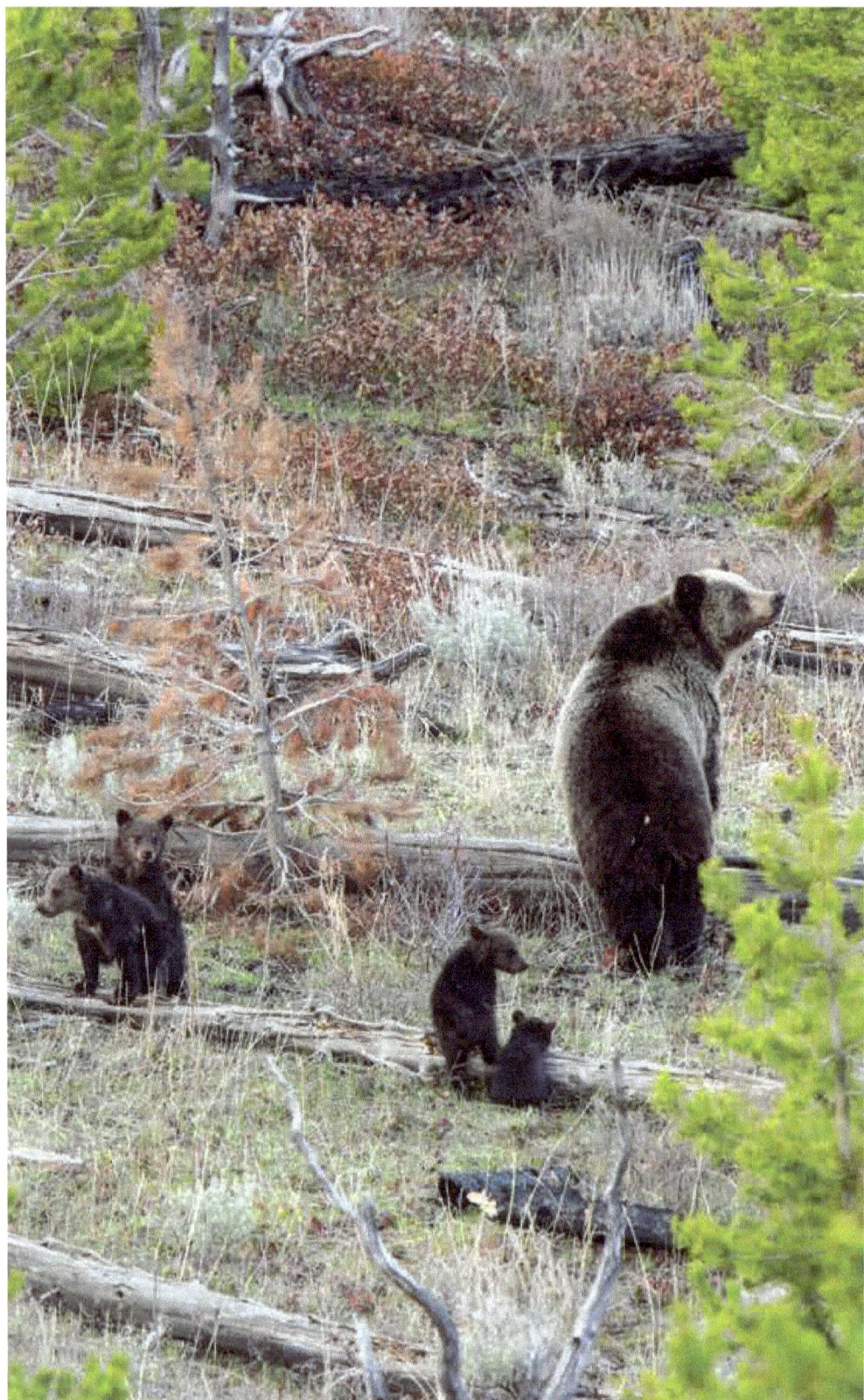

At least three of **Griz**zly 399's cubs are **docu**mented to have been killed by **hu**mans. One of her cubs, **Sno**wy, was struck by a car in Grand **Te**ton **Na**tional Park, while **an**other one, #615 was killed by a deer **hunt**er just **out**side the park's **safe**ty.

Human en**cro**achment in the **Pa**cific Creek **area** re**sul**ted in #587 **be**ing **re**moved from the **area** he grew up in and **re**located to the **Up**per Green **Riv**er. He **end**ed up **kill**ing **cat**tle and was **sub**sequently killed by the **Wyo**ming Fish & Game.

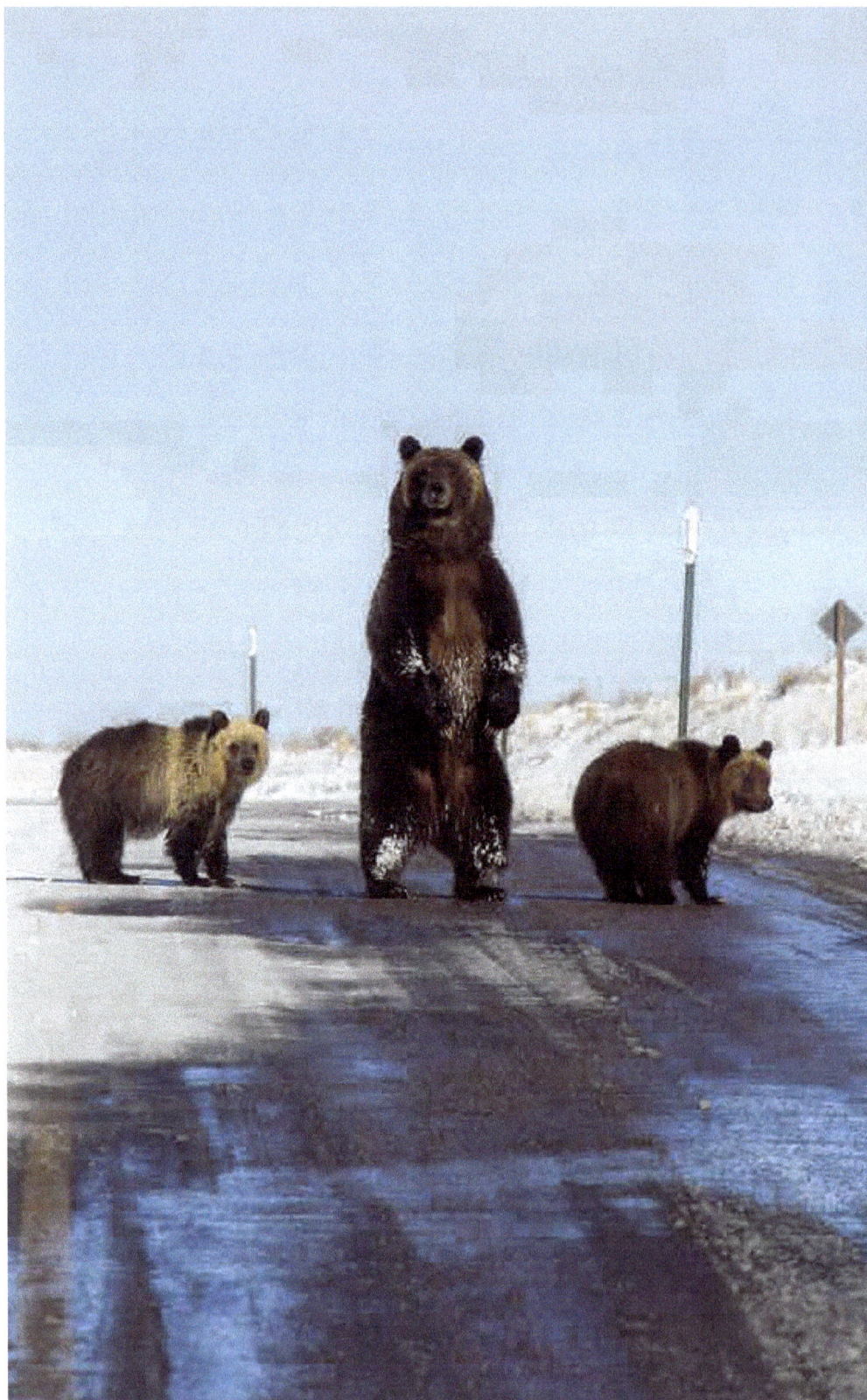

Unfortu**nately**, **Griz**zly 399 lost more of her cubs d**u**e to **neg**ative **im**pacts from **hu**mans. One of her four cubs, kn**o**wn as #1057, was **eu**tha**nized af**ter **re**p**ea**ted**ly **en**ter**ing res**iden**tial **ar**eas in the **Up**per Gr**ee**n **Riv**er in **Wy**o**ming**. The death of 1057 could have been **pr**e**vent**ed had p**eo**ple **se**c**u**red food **att**ract**ants a**round their h**o**mes.

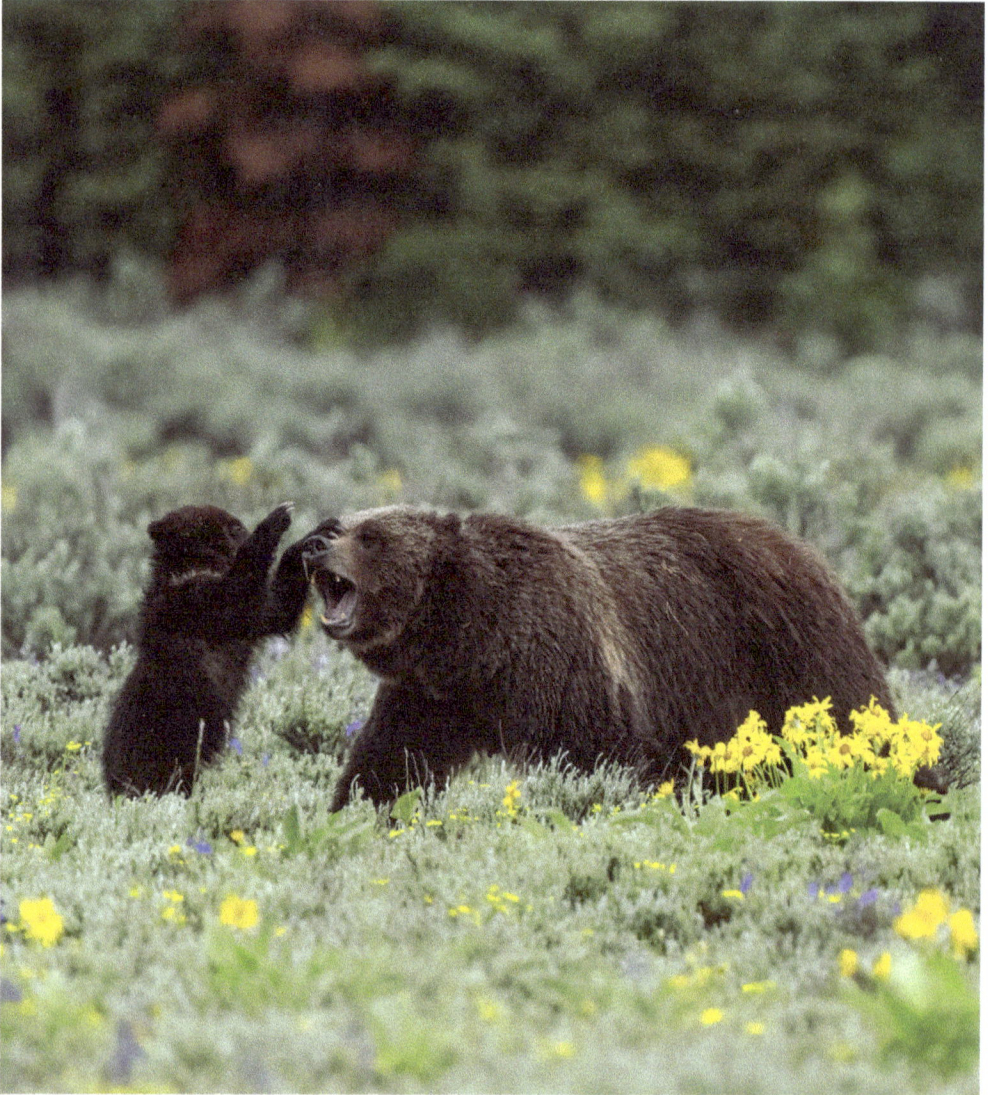

What is the **Sta**tus of **Griz**zly 399?

The **stor**y of **Griz**zly 399's has **cap**tiv**a**ted **man**y, **turn**ing her **in**to a **ce**leb**r**ity be**a**r. This **pop**u**lar**ity has **in**sp**i**red **doc**u**men**tary films, **nu**mer**ous** **ar**ticles, **a**dult and **chil**dren's books, and **e**ven her **o**wn **Face**book P**a**ge.

On M**a**y 16, 2023, **Griz**zly 399 **e**merged from **hi**bern**a**tion with a **beau**tiful cub, **lat**er kn**o**wn as **Spir**it. At the **a**ge 26 or 27, sh**e** **be**c**a**me the **old**est kn**o**wn **griz**zly be**a**r to have cubs in the **Grea**ter **Yel**l**o**w**sto**ne Ec**o**sys**tem** (**GY**E).

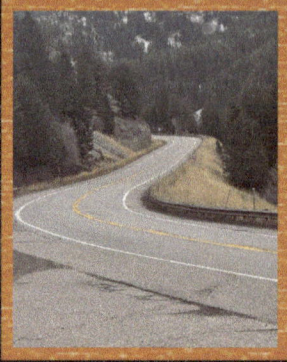

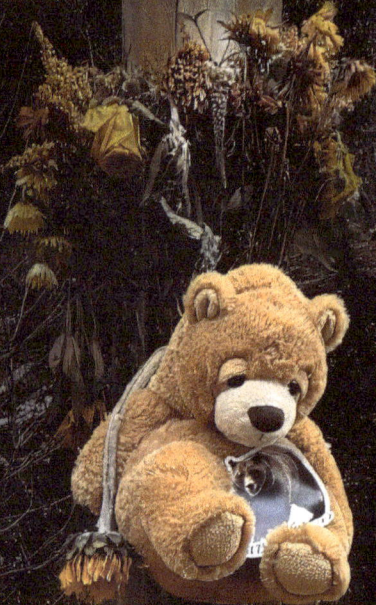

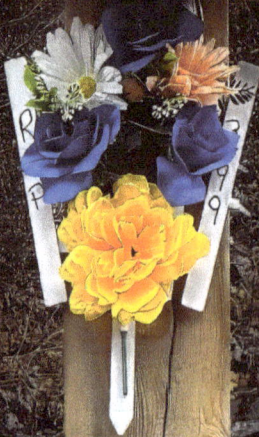

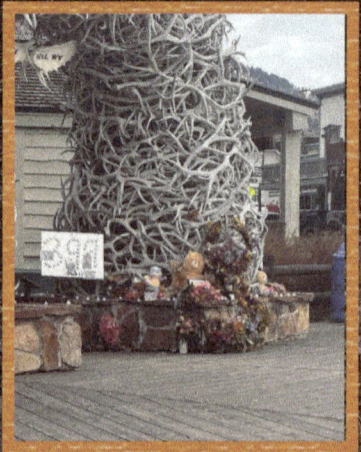

Tragically, on **Oct**o**ber** 22, 2024, while **Griz**zly 399 and her cub were **trav**el**ing a**long a road in the Snake River **Can**yon, the **moth**er bear was struck and killed by a car. **Spir**it **sur**vived and **hope**ful**ly** found her way back to **Te**ton **Na**tional Park.

There is hope that **Griz**zly 399's death will not be in vain; the State of **Wy**o**ming** is **con**sid**er**ing **ex**pand**ing** the **num**ber of **wild**life **cross**ings such as overpasses, **un**der**pass**es, and **cul**verts to **re**duce **wild**life-**ve**hicle hits.

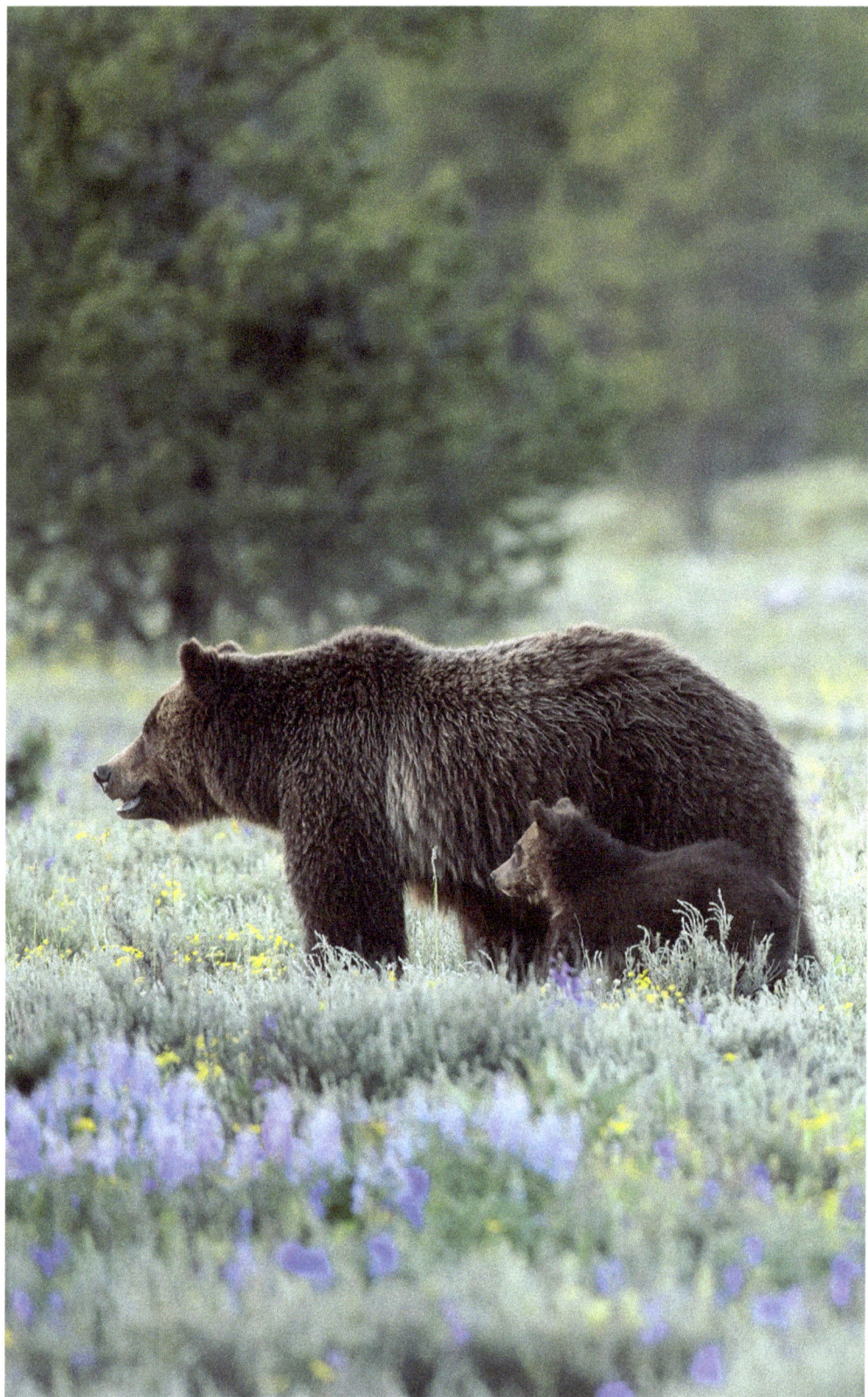

Grizzly Be<u>a</u>r Facts

- **Griz**zly **n<u>o</u>s**es are dished with a curve.
- **Griz**zly be<u>a</u>rs have short round <u>e</u>ars.
- **Griz**zli<u>e</u>s have a **sh<u>ou</u>l**der hump d<u>u</u>e to the **mas**sive **mus**cles in their **sh<u>ou</u>l**ders.
- **Griz**zly be<u>a</u>r fur **col**or **v<u>a</u>r**ies: Blond, **Red-**dish, **Gr<u>a</u>y**ish, and L<u>i</u>ght to Dark Brown. The l<u>i</u>ght tips on the ends of their fur **cre<u>a</u>**te what is called the "**griz**zled" look or blond str<u>e</u>aks on the be<u>a</u>rs.**Griz**zly 399 is **red**dish-brown.

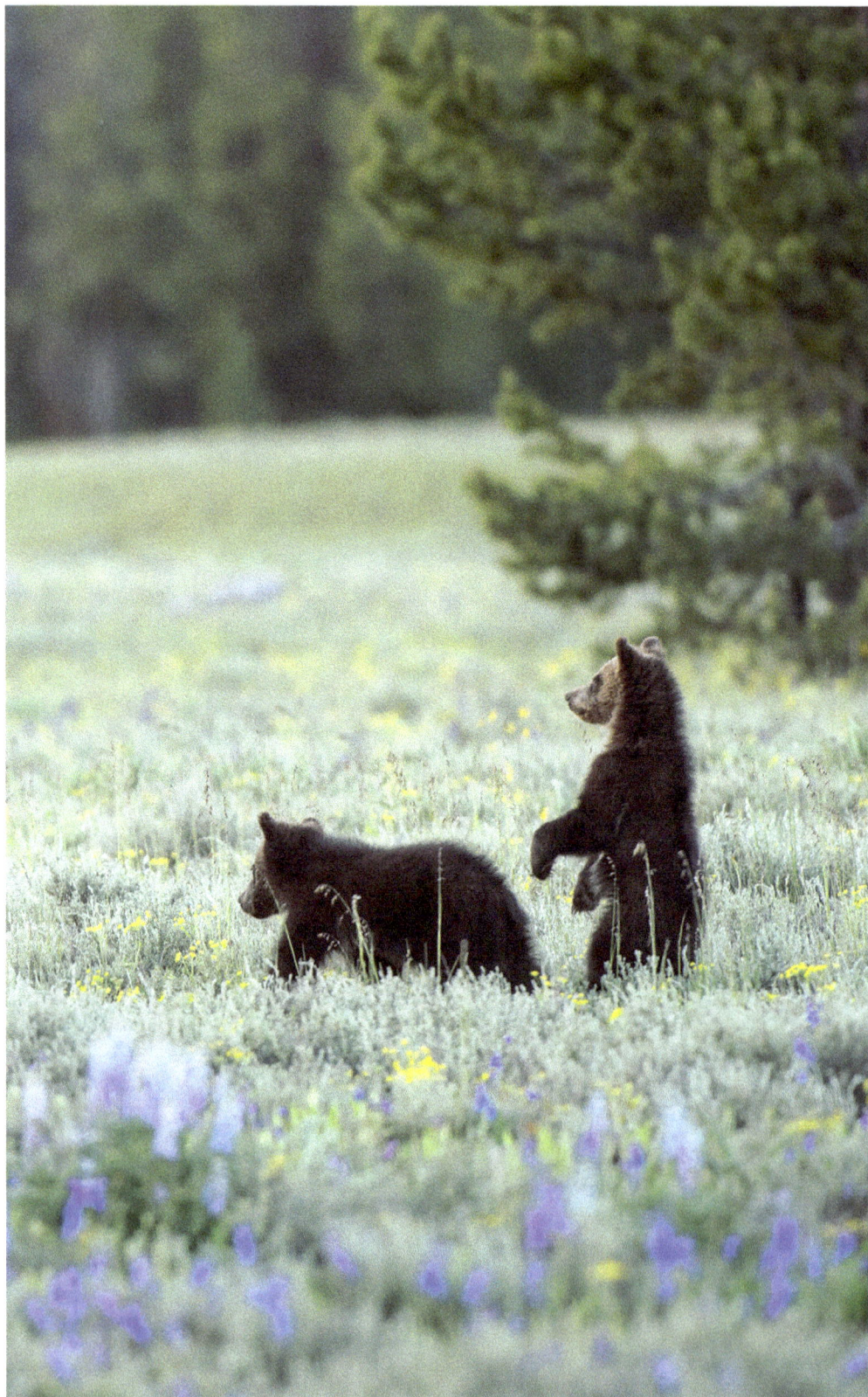

- **Griz**zly be<u>a</u>rs are **om**niv**or**ous - they <u>e</u>at **ber**ri<u>es</u>, **grass**es, **flow**ers, **tu**bers, w<u>i</u>ld **veg**gi<u>es</u>, **white**bark p<u>i</u>ne s<u>ee</u>ds, bugs, **fun**g<u>i</u>, fish, **ro**dents, **bi**son, elk, and dead **an**i**mals**.
- They <u>e</u>at up to 100 lbs. of food a d<u>a</u>y to store fat **re**serves to m<u>a</u>ke it thro<u>u</u>gh the long **win**ter.
- **Griz**zly be<u>a</u>r claws are 2" to 4" (5 to 10 cm) long. They are **sl<u>i</u>ght**ly curved and are **fre**quent**ly** <u>u</u>sed for **dig**ging foods or dens.
- **Griz**zly be<u>a</u>rs have 1 to 4 cubs per birth but **typ**ical**l**y have twins or **tri**plets.
- The cubs are bl<u>i</u>nd, **tooth**less, and **h<u>ai</u>r**less when they are born **dur**ing the **win**ter.

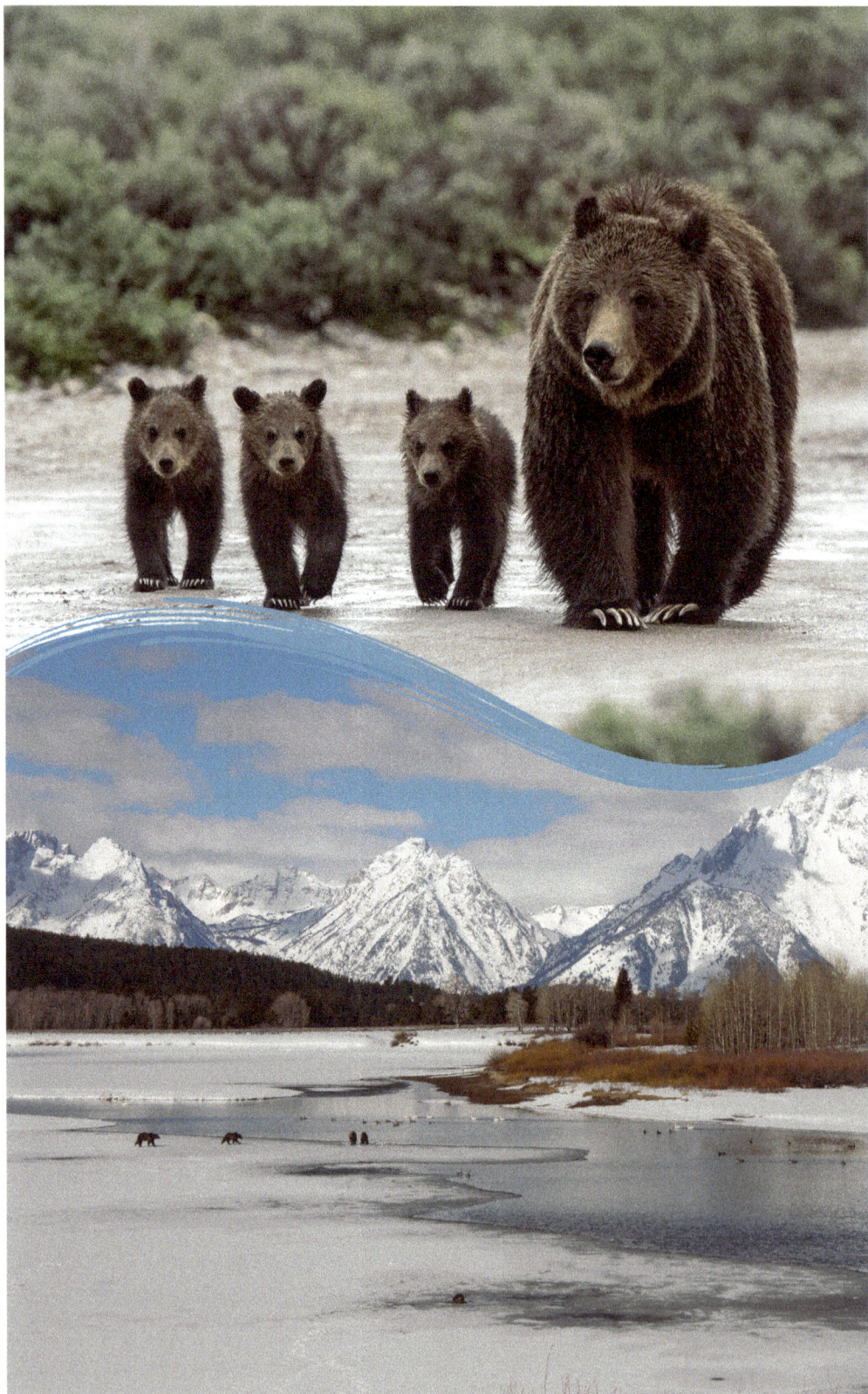

Grizzly be**a**rs are **essential** in **for**est
ec**o**sys**tems be**cause:

- They are s**ee**d **spread**ers, **pass**ing them
through their **bod**i**es** as **fer**til**i**zed s**ee**ds.
- When **scav**eng**ing**, be**a**rs dig up the soil,
helping to cr**ea**te n**i**trogen-rich soil.
- **No**ta**bly**, **griz**zli**es** **reg**ul**ate** prey
popul**a**tions and **pre**vent **o**ver**graz**ing

Roughly 60,000 **griz**zli**es** live in the
Uni**ted** St**a**tes and **Can**ada, with more than
half in **A**las**ka**.

In the **low**er 48 st**a**tes, there are
approxim**a**tely 1,900 **griz**zli**es**, thanks to
the **En**d**a**n**gered Spe**ci**es** Act.

In the **Grea**ter **Yell**ow**stone E**c**o**sys**tem,
the **griz**zly be**a**r **pop**ul**a**tion has been:

350 bears in 1975	737 bears in 2019
757 bears in 2014	1,063 bears in 2021
712 bears in 2018	1,030 bears in 2023

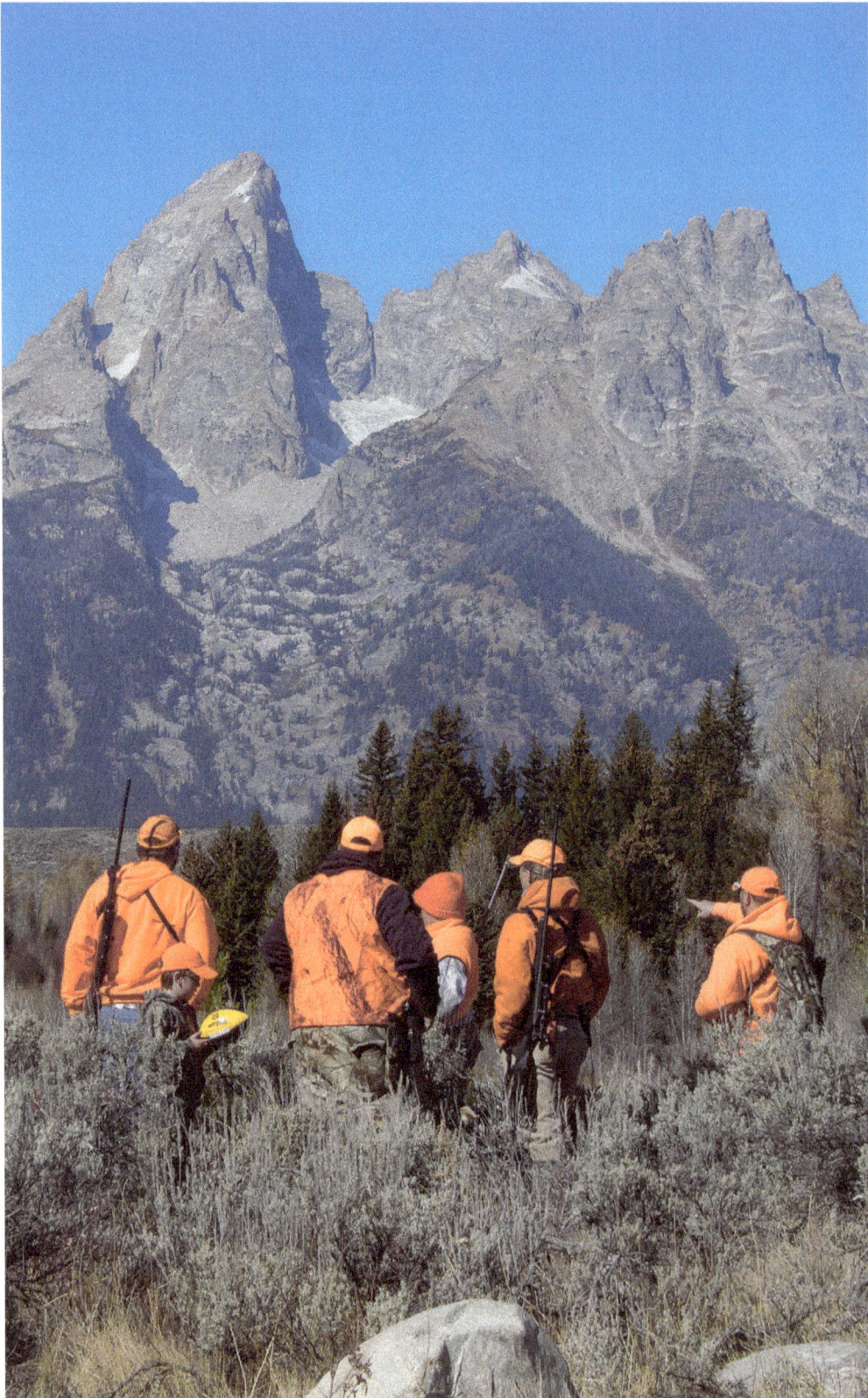

Negative Impacts From Human Interaction

- **Automobile accidents**: **Grizzly** bear deaths as they cross the road.
- **Habituation**: **Grizzlies** search for **eas**y food such as **unsecured gar**bage, **camp**er's food and **ref**use, or **road**kill.
- **Hunt**ing: **During** the **annual** elk hunt in Grand **Teton National** Park and the **surrounding Bridger Teton National Forest, grizzlies** learn to **associate** the sound of **gun**shots with food and seek out the **car**cass. Their **pres**ence in the **hunt**ing area may **create conflict.**

These types of **interactions** bring bears close to **hu**mans and cause **potential conflict.** When this **hap**pens, the bear is trapped, **sedated,** ear-tagged, **radio**-collared, and **relocat**ed to **unfamil**iar **habitat** or may be killed.

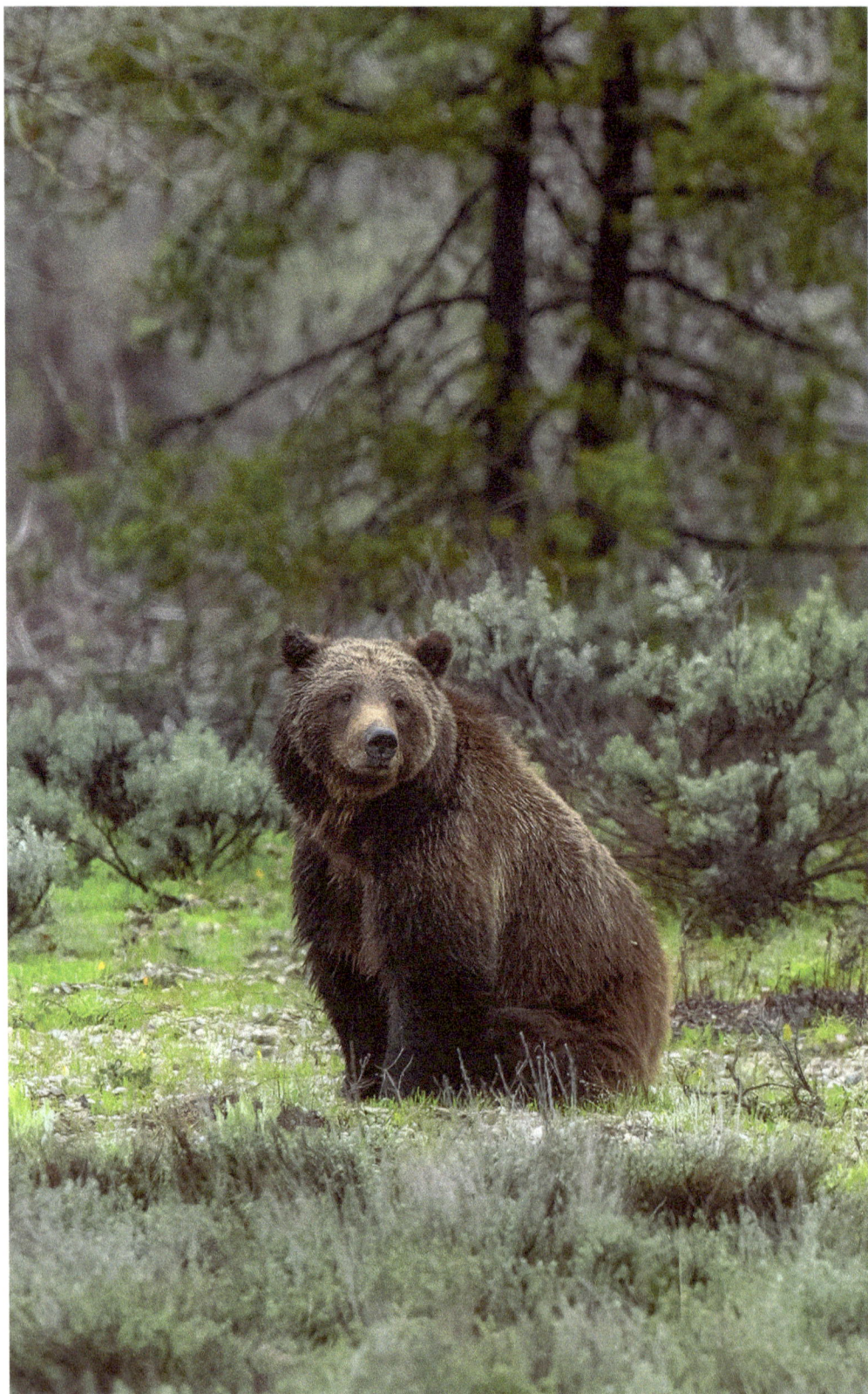

Climate Change and its Impact on Grizzly Bear Survival

Due to **global** **warm**ing, pine **bee**tles are **flourishing** at **high**er **eleva**tions, **kill**ing **white**bark pine trees. The high-fat seeds of **white**bark pine are **critical** food for **Yellowstone griz**zlies, **es**pe**cial**ly **fe**males that **pro**duce more cubs when seeds are **a**bun**dant**. A non-**na**tive **fun**gus, white pine **blis**ter rust, is **also kill**ing **white**bark pine.

Other **im**pacts: **Cut**throat trout have been an **impor**tant food for **griz**zlies. **Be**cause non-**na**tive Lake Trout were **il**le**gal**ly **intro**duced **in**to **Yel**low**stone** Lake. These fish preyed on the **Cut**throat trout, **dras**tically **re**duc**ing** their **num**bers.

As a **conse**quence of this **de**cline, **griz**zly bears are **seek**ing food **clos**er to **hu**man **settlements, lead**ing to an **in**crease in **con**flicts **be**tween bears and **peo**ple.

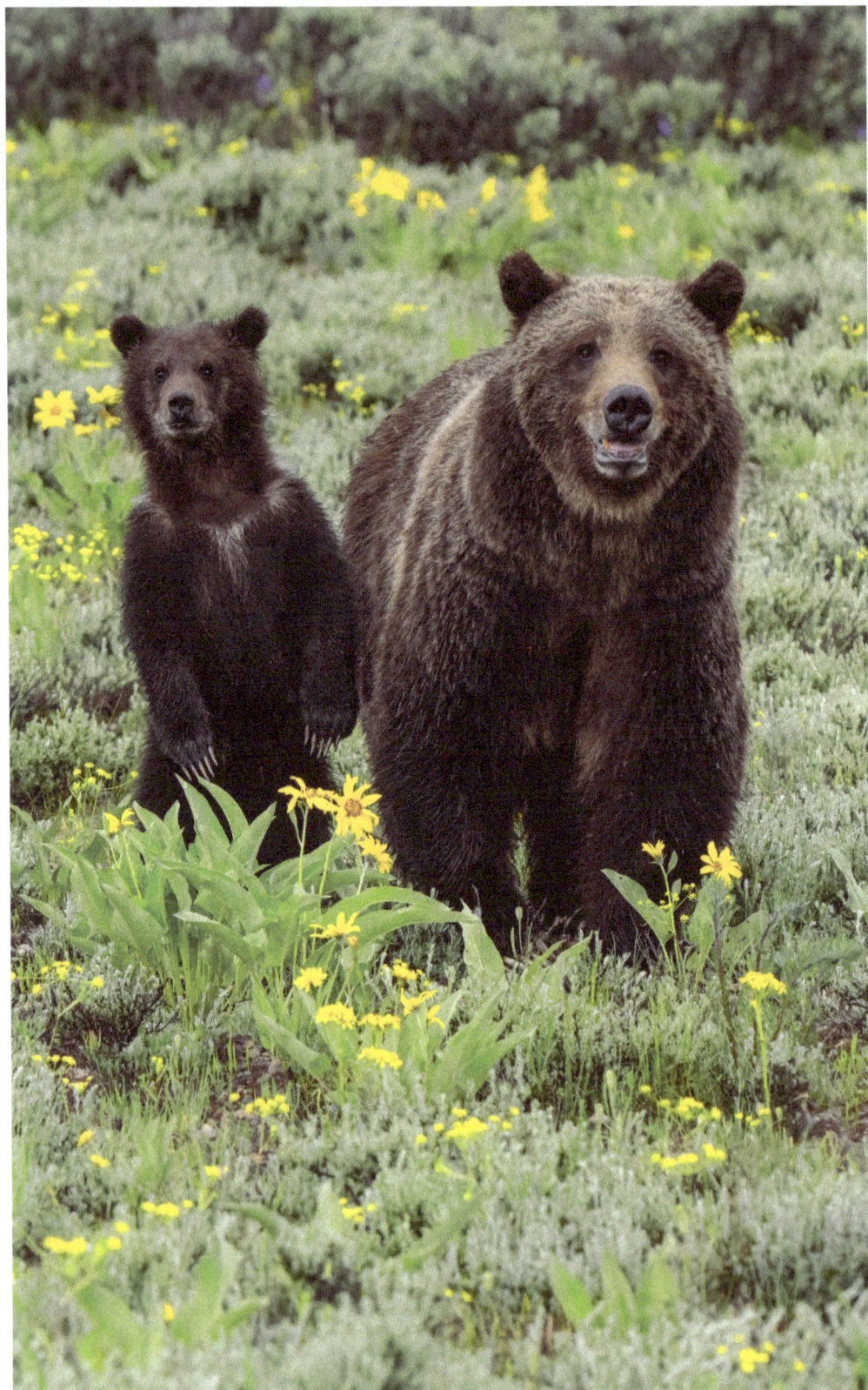

Grizzli<u>e</u>s r<u>e</u>quire **sufficient ter**rito<u>rie</u>s to live, but their **hab**itats are **shrink**ing d<u>u</u>e to **hu**man **en**cr<u>o</u>ach**ment**.

The f<u>u</u>ture **ef**fects of **cli**mate ch<u>a</u>nge on the **griz**zly be<u>a</u>r r<u>e</u>m<u>a</u>in **large**ly **un**kn<u>o</u>wn.

But a **bet**ter **un**der**stand**ing of th<u>e</u>se **mag**nificent **animals** are **nec**ess<u>a</u>ry for their **sur**v<u>i</u>**val**.

W<u>e</u> n<u>ee</u>d to **a**dopt **com**pas**sion** and **tole**rance **to**wards **griz**zli<u>e</u>s more than **ev**er as they **a**dapt to a **chang**ing world.

Dedicated to Thomas D. Mangelsen and all those who work tirelessly to protect bears like Grizzly 399 so that our children and grandchildren can enjoy these majestic animals in the future.

It is essential that we all appreciate, respect, and educate ourselves about the value of these magnificent bears!

- Sylvia M. Medina

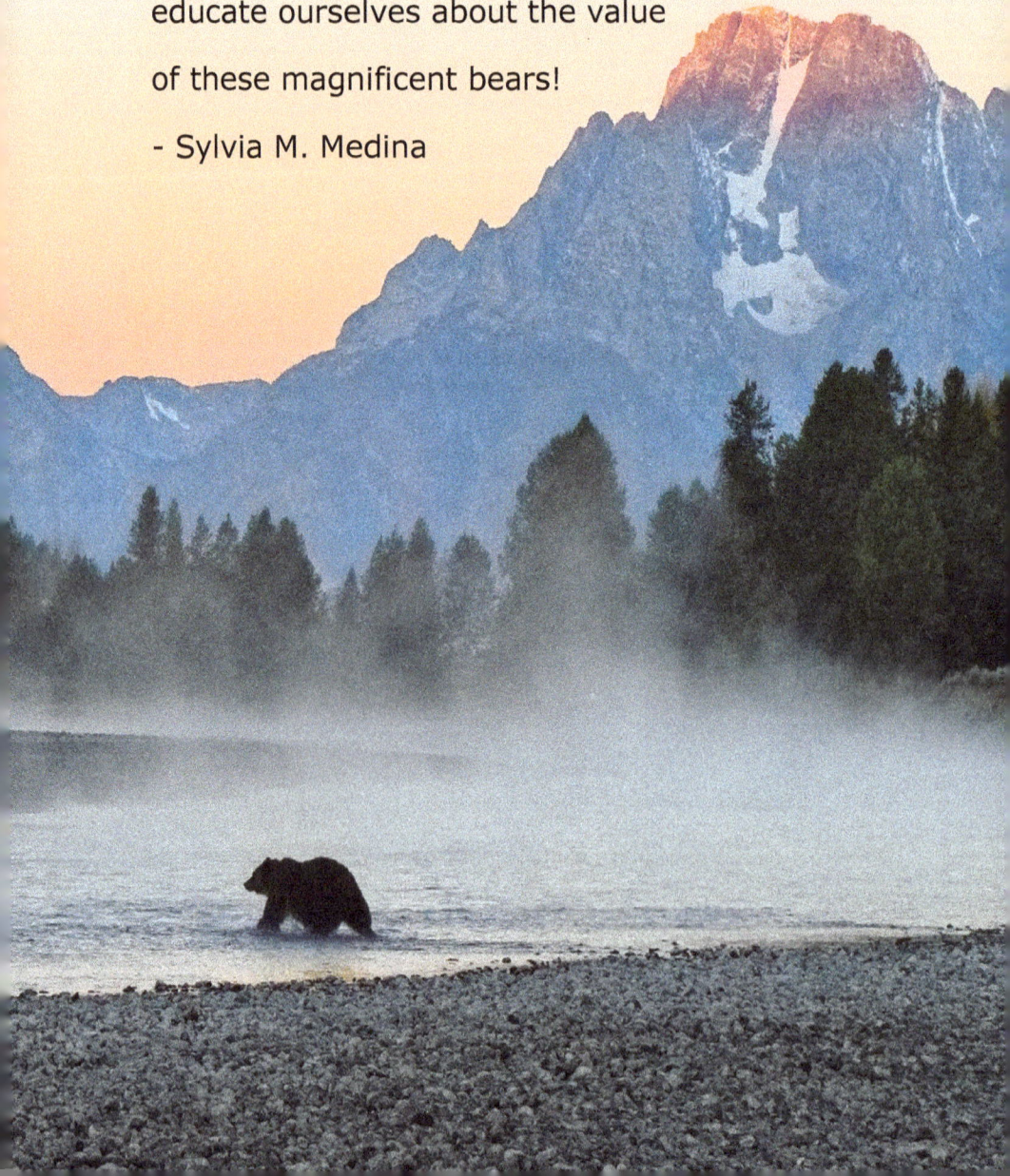

The following organizations contribute to saving animals and our world.

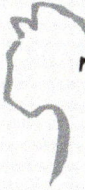

THE COUGAR FUND

The Cougar Fund was founded in 2001
by writer Cara Blessley Lowe and
photographer Thomas D. Mangelsen
after a firsthand experience observing a
mother lion they named "Spirit" and her
three cubs on the National Elk Refuge in
Jackson Hole, Wyoming.
cougarfund.org

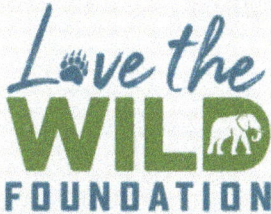

Love the WILD FOUNDATION

Love The Wild Foundation empowers children around the world to appreciate their local resources and ecosystems, to understand their connectivity to regional and global resources and ecosystems, and how to protect them.

Sound K<u>e</u>y

How Noah Text® Works

Noah Text® allows readers to see sound-parts within words, providing a way for struggling readers to decode and enunciate words that are difficult to access. In turn, their improvement in reading accuracy and fluency frees up cognitive resources that they can devote to comprehending the meaning of the text, enabling them to truly enjoy reading while building their reading skills.

Syllables

A *syllable* is a unit of pronunciation with only one vowel sound, with or without surrounding consonants. Syllables line up with the way we speak and are an integrated unit of speech and hearing. Teachers often clap out syllables with their students.

Noah Text® acts upon words with more than one syllable. In a multiple-syllable word, the presentation of each syllable alternates bold, not bold, bold, etc. For example, the word "syllable" would be presented as "**syl**la**ble**," while the word "sound" is not changed at all.

Vowels

A long vowel is a vowel that pronounces its own letter name. Here are some examples of underlined long vowels you will find in Noah Text®, along with syllable breaks that are made obvious:

Long (a)

pl<u>a</u>te, p<u>ai</u>n, **hes**i**t<u>a</u>te**, **n<u>a</u>**tion

h<u>ai</u>r, r<u>a</u>re, **par**ent, **l<u>i</u>**br<u>a</u>ry

p<u>a</u>le, f<u>ai</u>l, **de**t<u>ai</u>l

tr<u>a</u>y, **al**w<u>a</u>ys

Long (e)

feet, teach, **com**plete

feel, deal, **ap**peal

ear, fear, here, **dis**ap**pear**, **se**vere

Long (i)

tribe, like, night, **high**light

fire, **ad**mire, **re**quire

mile, pile, **a**while, **rep**tile

Long (o)

globe, nose, **sup**pose, **re**mote

coach, whole, coal, goal, **ap**proach

mow, blown, **win**dow

Long (u)

huge, mule, **fu**el, **per**fume, **a**muse

hue, **ar**gue, **tis**sue, blue, **pol**lution

Disclaimer: As noted in the research provided at noahtext.com, the English writing system is extremely complex. Thus, the process of segmenting syllables, identifying rime patterns, and highlighting long vowels, is not only tedious but ambiguous at times based on the pronunciation of various regional dialects, the complexity of English orthography, and other articulatory considerations. Noah Text® strives to be as accurate as possible in developing clear, concise modified text that will assist readers; however, it cannot guarantee universal agreement on how all words are pronounced.

www.ingramcontent.com/pod-product-compliance
Lightning Source LLC
Chambersburg PA
CBHW040907210326
41597CB00029B/4999